THE MYSTERY THAT BINDS ME STILL

By Mickie R. Singer

'One million people commit suicide every year'
The World Health Organization

Mickie R. Singer

Published by
Chipmunkapublishing
PO Box 6872
Brentwood
Essex CM13 1ZT
United Kingdom

http://www.chipmunkapublishing.com

Edited by Linda Zamboglou

THE MYSTERY THAT BINDS ME STILL

FOR DAN

Mickie R. Singer

THE MYSTERY THAT BINDS ME STILL

Alone

From childhood's hour I have not been
As others were; I have not seen
As others saw; I could not bring
My passions from a common spring.
From the same source I have not taken
My sorrow; I could not awaken
My heart to joy at the same tone;
And all I loved, I loved alone.
Then – in my childhood, in the dawn
Of a stormy life – was drawn
From every depth of good and ill
The mystery that binds me still:
From the torrent, or the fountain,
From the red cliff of the mountain,
From the sun that round me, I rolled
In its autumn tint of gold,
From the lightning in the sky
As it passed me flying by,
From the thunder and the storm,
And the cloud that took the form
(When the rest of Heaven was blue)
Of a demon in my view.

By Edgar Allan Poe

Mickie R. Singer

THE MYSTERY THAT BINDS ME STILL

PREFACE

I am Mack Singer's daughter. Most likely you would not recognize his name. He was neither famous nor rich nor known to the public. Nonetheless, he was legendary.

My story begins with him.

My father and his life were both dramatic. He made his living as an upholsterer but shone as an actor. His stage was confined to Cincinnati, in a group called the Bureau Players and in early television at station WKRC. The author of those shows was a young Rod Serling, later writer and narrator of the television series, "The Twilight Zone." Originating over forty years ago, it is so popular it's still in reruns today. Being a man touched by magic, it was only fitting that Rod Serling became Dad's good friend.

Dad was given to quoting some of his oddest old lines at the most unexpected times. I once dropped a bowl of mashed potatoes because he had unnerved me with his sudden shouting: "By the bones of Hallibar! By the bones of Hallibar!" thundering from his mouth.

My father was a believer in the little people, whom he defined as the fairies and the leprechauns. He taught me how to look for them. You couldn't see them if you looked for them straight ahead, he'd tell me. "You've gotta look slaunchwise," he said. Looking slaunchwise involved holding your head very still while you raised your eyebrows and slid your eyes north and south. He never saw them but he was ready for them, and that, he told me, is what counts.

Fantasy was very important to my father. During his bitter childhood, tales of alternative worlds in early science fiction and fantasy magazines gave him sanctuary and hope. One story in particular stayed with him through the years. It featured nine invisible gods that sat on a man's shoulders and kept him safe. Dad borrowed these gods for his own. At thirty he met a curly-haired woman with "bedroom" eyes. He wanted to marry her only a few days after they met. But first she had to pass the test.

Dad told my future mother he had nine invisible gods that sat on his shoulders and when she didn't so much as flinch he was sure she was meant for him. On the tenth day of their courtship he asked her to marry him, and several months later, he and Jean May Rukin were wed. They had a small ceremony with a justice of the peace, inviting a few family members and friends. Afterwards my grandmother had a reception at her house. Late in the afternoon my father announced he was tired and he was by God going to bed and taking his wife with him. If anyone wanted to see them they'd have to come to the bedroom. Several of their friends complied, chewing on tuna fish sandwiches while being entertained by the pajama-d newlyweds.

Meeting my mother was the best thing that ever happened to my father. Not only was everything before that prologue, it was hell.

THE MYSTERY THAT BINDS ME STILL

My father might have been born in 1909. No one, including my father, knew for sure. Dad never had a birthday or been told his age. His birth records burned up in a fire in his former hometown. When he met Mom he selected August 15th as his day. From then on his birthday was celebrated with Mom making his favorite foods, "Eggplant Repulsive" and "Smashed Lima Beans." My brothers and I always dreaded it. Though I admired my father greatly, I must admit I didn't always care for his taste.

Mom's absolute priority was Dad, the care and feeding thereof. Dad's priority was letting her do it. It seemed to work. They were married and in love for 53 years.

Dad's father was a hops farmer somewhere in the Georgian region of Russia. Dad had several brothers and one sister. I'm not sure how many brothers he had, because several of them were killed in pogroms. Besides Louis and Will, only the name "Sholom" remains in my head. They were Jews, and Jews in Russia were a: poor and b: isolated from their Christian neighbors. My father's family was neither, owing to the Russian thirst for beer.

I will not refer to my father's father as my grandfather. Dad would be most upset if I did. He insisted that "that man" was no father of his. I had strict instructions never to so much as suggest I was related to him. Dad would literally growl at the thought. Biologically he was unquestionably Dad's father. Although I never met him I saw a picture of him once. He looked exactly like Dad. This was extremely ironic because the reason you-know-who hated my father was because he didn't believe Dad was his.

My grandmother Freida (I *am* allowed to claim *her*) was in fact a faithful wife but her husband didn't return the sentiment. He regularly transported escaping Jews in his wagon under the hops. He'd bribe the border guards to let him pass. Apparently he was very generous because a loyal guard let him know one night that he had been discovered. The Cossacks were on their way to take him to jail when he escaped and eventually came to America, settling in Philadelphia, where he promptly and illegally took another wife.

While he began a new life his son Sholom was murdered during a pogrom; the Cossacks conscripted Lou to be in the Russian Army for 25 years and when he escaped, a soldier slit his throat from end to end. Amazingly, Lou survived and eventually he, Will's sister Sophie and Freida all came to America. They tracked down you-know-who in Philadelphia.

But he refused to have anything to do with them.

In 1914 both Freida and my father fell ill during the Spanish flu epidemic. The hospitals were too full to take them in, but the nuns did. Thus began my father's lifelong emotional attachment to Catholicism. Heartbroken, he watched his mother die in the bed next to him. He was left with nowhere to go but to you-know-who's house, and his hate.

THE MYSTERY THAT BINDS ME STILL

In the early twentieth century the word "abuse" wasn't applied to what some endured behind closed doors. Nonetheless, you-know-who employed every possible form of verbal, mental and physical abuse toward my father, regularly making use of clubs and whips. According to Dad, the result was that he became a turn-of-the century juvenile delinquent, a hardened, tough "little son of a bitch."

This was perhaps best illustrated by my father's actions when you-know-who sent him to a rabbi to learn Hebrew. This particular rabbi was also abusive. He used a short whip to "correct" his students when they were wrong.

During one session Dad decided he had had enough. He grabbed the whip out of the rabbi's hand and chased him around the table, giving the rabbi a sharp taste of his own methods. He did not go back again.

Dad grew up wild in South Philly's streets. He wasn't particularly obedient in school either, but he was smart. He never made less than an "A." Although he left school at the age of 14, he knew 6 different languages, having picked them up from the various ethnic groups he grew up with. For the rest of his life he would regret his lack of formal education. His original desire was to be a librarian. He was a voracious reader, going to the library weekly and polishing off several books. When he was in his seventies he and Mom enrolled in college at the University of California in Long Beach. Dad specialized in Native American studies and was formally adopted by the Pima

Indian tribe. He was made a group instructor in one of his classes and found himself actually teaching – and loving it. Both he and Mom became ESL instructors as well.

Perhaps his bitterest memory was of you-know-who taking him to an orphanage at the age of ten. You-know-who actually tried to bribe the directors to take Dad. But they turned him down. So both of them came back home; neither of them happy about it.

At 14 Dad ran away from home and never returned, drifting across the country. Because he needed a trade he chose upholstery. He took care to be good at it. He was a great believer in the idea that if you're going to do something, do it well. In Cincinnati he developed an impressive enough reputation that he did upholstery work for the most posh department stores and for some of the museums. One time – don't ask me how, I was too young to know – he upholstered Liberace's furniture. The whole family was particularly amused by Liberace's throne chair. Just like his clothes, it was over-the-top: grandiose with gold paint and red velvet – and at the end of each of the arms, where one would rest one's hands – there were two enormous golden breasts.

Becoming an upholsterer helped Dad find a perfect place to express his rage. When he became active in the upholsterer's union he quite literally fought for union rights in the streets, battling bosses, strikebreakers and police. He was fond of pointing to a bump on his nose and saying "See this? This is from a lead pipe." His street fighting resulted in numerous stays in prison. He never told me how many times or for how long. All he said was "*I was never in jail.*" Apparently he used various aliases but not his real name.

Even my father's legal name was an alias too. Coming from Russia his name was "Avrom Hersh Tzintz." The immigration officials at Ellis Island quickly changed it to "Abraham Harry Singer." Their decisions, at the time, were law. Dad was best known by his nicknames, which were in turn variations of "Mox" "Little Mox" and "Max." Later on when he had to apply for citizenship he had to pick a name and stay with it. "Mack Harry Singer" was his choice.

The citizenship problem was a sticky one. Dad thought he *was* a citizen. You-know-who had said he'd gotten his citizenship papers, so all the children were U.S. citizens as well. After Mom and Dad had married and had two children his lack of actual citizenship came to light. He was threatened with deportment. During his hearing Dad had to prove he had a record of law-abiding behavior. This was a considerable fly in the ointment. How he managed to get past it, I am lifelong bound not to say.

Not only had he been in jail, he'd associated in many nefarious activities as well. He told me about a prostitute he'd once known (he didn't say how) who asked him to be her pimp – which he declined. Dad was also given several different nicknames during his years of traveling. One of them was "LotsaPoppa." I declined to ask him why.

It was clear, however, that during that time he hated his own Judaism. He associated it with his father and the abusive rabbi. But he felt safe and protected with Catholics because of the nuns having taken him in. For years Dad socialized exclusively with Irish or Italian Catholics. He picked up a passion for olives and leprechauns and became the only Russian Jew to maintain hailed from County Cork.

Dad never converted but he was confused, and he raised me to be equally so. On one hand he was staunchly Jewish but on the other he refused to go to Temple. He was quite comfortable, however, with my attending mass at St. Agnes. On Christmas Eve the whole family watched Midnight Mass on television, but we never had stockings or a Christmas tree. Mom tried to install some Jewish identification in us. She made a fairly big deal out of Passover and Chanukah and lighting the candles for Sabbath dinner (until she began to fear that our bird would fly into the flame.) Dad, however, would grumble outrageously anti-Semitic remarks like "Never be in a room with more than three Jews at a time." Yet when Joey Bishop or some other Jewish comedian would show up on a television show he'd yell "Jew boy!" and beam with pride that a Jew had made it big.

Go figure.

I couldn't decide whether I was Jewish or Catholic, Irish or Italian. At one point in my childhood I contemplated giving up on the whole thing and becoming a Protestant. But I couldn't pull it off. There was a tiny dose of Judaism that had crept into my soul. It took hold, albeit dim and faint.

Dad was wonderfully mild-mannered and loving. In later years friends called him "Kindly Old Philosopher." When asked how he was, he would always say, "I'm breathing. Life is good." The love he found in Mom and his kids erased that sad "little son of a bitch" - except when he was mad. Dad's temper was legendary too.

My father's years in the streets had affected him deeply. Touch one of his hidden triggers and he'd turn instantly furious, vengeful and mean. It didn't happen often but when it did it was horrific. He told me that when he became angry he literally saw red, and I believe it was true. His voice could take on a tone that would scare the poop out of an elephant. From the time he left Philadelphia he always carried a switchblade in his pocket with his hand inside, ready to fight. It was somewhat unnerving walking with Dad to the library, which seemed in our quiet neighborhood a pretty safe thing to do. Nonetheless he'd have his hand deep in his pocket, alert for danger; all systems go to brandish the knife. He kept a crowbar on his night table, ready to do battle with burglars. He also kept a gun in one of his dresser drawers. One night a severely intoxicated young man pounded on our door at 2 a.m., demanding to be let in. In his inebriated state, he apparently thought our house was where he lived. Immediately, Dad was at the doorway with his gun. Pre-911, I was frantically begging the operator to call the police. I wasn't particularly scared that this befuddled fellow would break in; I was terrified Dad was going to shoot him.

There were family stories of Dad threatening people but I never saw him do so - they happened before I was born. When my brother Jon was a little boy he almost got run over by a truck. My father was witness to this. Immediately he pulled out his knife and ran toward the truck, pounding on the door. The driver speedily rolled up his windows and sped off.

In another incident, Dad got angry at a co-worker and went after him with a pair of scissors. He was prevented from doing murder only because he was held back by his fellow employees.

Yet few who knew this mild-mannered, good-hearted man would believe he ever displayed such behavior as that.

To Dad's credit he mellowed considerably as his life went on, although he never took his hand off of his knife. I was the child who most received his gentleness and sweet nature. I was his princess, his little girl. He made me feel special. He encouraged every aspect of my imagination. Together we wove stories. Sometimes I'd come down to the basement where he kept his shop and I'd tell him a tale while he worked. At bedtimes if he didn't read to me from the Oz books we would build "story trees." They were made of stories, with branches we'd pretend to be made of a different candy every night. No matter whose turn it was, he reserved the right at the end to have the top branch. This was always covered with "a thick white blanket of sour cream."

I still think sour cream is the greatest thing there is.

Dad was simply larger than life. He was immensely funny, given to popping off whimsical comments at any given time. I recall with fondness his telling Mom to "excuse my entire face." Another one of my favorites was when my mother yelled at him for packing peanut butter cups into a picnic lunch already bulging with food. "We've got enough food for an army!" she snapped. In his characteristic mildness Dad replied "But this is for the Navy."

He was never without an opinion or political passion. He was a deeply righteous man who cared about what he felt was right and he was willing to do what it took to make it so. Despite his adventures in the streets, or perhaps because of them, Dad had solid Judeo-Christian values and beliefs. He was absolutely insistent that his children have the same. The worst thing we could do was to be rude or thoughtless toward someone or to show up late. "You have to respect people's time," he insisted. He taught my brothers to be gentlemen, demanding at dinnertime they pull Mom's chair out for her and push it gently back. God help you if you did anything that upset Mom. Dad was her champion, her loyal white knight.

Most of all, my father loved people. He gloried in them. He loved to watch them, to appreciate the things they said and did. People flocked to him, attracted by his humor and warmth.

Later in his life Dad kept journals where he wrote down his observations. When he observed a random act of kindness or overheard a conversation that amused him, he'd write it down. One of my favorite entries was written after he came out of the hospital for a hip operation. A concerned neighbor asked him "How are you, Mr. Singer?" Dad replied, "I'm bursting with euphoria!" "Oh dear," she replied. "Does it hurt?"

My father's influence guided my life. He believed in me, and told me so. "You can do anything you want to," he said, and so I believed it too. This was terribly important to me, in light of being most often in the charge of my mother, who suffered from untreated mental illness.

Mom had the misfortune of inheriting a long line of mental disorders, going back to at least my great grandmother and likely beyond. Growing up with a mentally ill mother didn't help matters. In the early 1900's few knew about mental illness, neither how to recognize nor treat it. She developed a host of symptoms, being highly stressed, depressed and afraid to leave her house. Mom thought she was an "emotional cripple." In her view, what she had was beyond being "crazy." It was something else, something even more sinister and threatening.

She was not a happy woman. Her face carried a permanent frown. As a result, it was only on occasion that I could experience the warm, funny and loving person she was. She was a talented artist and had once been a dancer. She was bright and well read and had a sense of humor under that groaning layer that burdened her so much of the time. She also had suicidal ideation and was given to writing me suicide notes. It was creepy to the utmost. Anger and criticism came easily and sometimes she was downright mean. Thus, Dad became the good guy, the one who appeared to believe in my dreams. Mom believed in smashing them. That was her way of "protecting" me from "the cruelty of life and its disappointments."

Even her tenderness could be quite disconcerting. When I was a little girl she told me not to worry about anything because after all, the roof could cave in any minute, so why fret? She thought she was comforting me. Instead, I started worrying I was going to be crushed by a falling ceiling.

Dad wasn't perfect, as a father or a man. There were times when he hurt me deeply. But he brought in the fairies, the magic, the hope and the light. He was the bright spark that gave me gumption. While Mom invited me into her fear, Dad encouraged me to celebrate life.

He may have molded me to be like him, but he wasn't necessarily prepared for what he would get. He wanted a rebel, but he found it hard to deal with me when I became more of a rebel than him. He encouraged me to be "different," but wasn't always comfortable with *how* different I could be. He hoped I'd stand up and be an individual, but found it hard to take my politics, rag-tag boyfriends and oddball friends.

Most of all, he wasn't prepared for his little princess to become more mentally ill than his wife. No one knew what was "wrong with me;" it was simply apparent early on that something was. During my worst episodes his ulcers rioted. He watched as I battled six different disorders which remained, for forty years, undiagnosed. He died before I had a diagnosis, appropriate treatment or medication. I can only imagine his pain.

I've been told I'm a walking miracle. I think that's stretching it a bit. I *have* managed to hold it together enough over the years to become a teacher, a storyteller, a writer and a college instructor. I have functioned during the slavery of rituals in severe OCD (obsessive compulsive disorder); and surfed the dizzying ups and downs of bi-polar disease. I inherited all of my mother's disorders and added on more of my own. Still, I've survived addictions, low self-esteem, an abusive marriage, single parenthood, and assorted other traumatic things. I have also inherited my father's gift of meeting life headstrong, stubborn and enjoying every moment that I can. I know that without my father's legacy, the gift of his fantasy, humor and determination, I would never have made it. Happily, I am still here today, neither crazy nor dead. Some days when I reflect on that, I am absolutely amazed.

I share a lot of characteristics with Dad. Like him, I like people, love to talk, hold grudges, tell stories, get angry, rebel against rules, value playmates, friendship and respect, converse with the fairies, enjoy being outrageous and stand up

THE MYSTERY THAT BINDS ME STILL

for what I believe. For good and for ill, I am Mack Singer's daughter. I tender my life a tribute to him.

The rest of this story will be mine rather than my Dad's. I have written this book hoping my experience can be healing or helpful for others. Some who read it might take heart when they discover they are not alone. Perhaps it will provide some inspiration or cheer. One of my favorite poets, Kenneth Patchen, wrote a book with a title that says it all: "Hallelujah Anyway." That is what this book is all about. The human spirit is incredibly strong – we can survive unspeakable horrors, and still celebrate, and still laugh. Sometimes it comes down to knowing that if you're breathing, life is good. For anyone who needs a reminder of that, I tender this book.

Mickie R. Singer

THE MYSTERY THAT BINDS ME STILL

CHAPTER ONE: IT BEGINS

Unlike David Copperfield, I am not yet born. My story begins with the family trauma that took place before I was here at all.

We were a family of three children, but I often felt like an afterthought and an only child. This was not just because my brothers were a great deal older than me, but because Mom, Dad, Barry and Jon had bonded together through a crisis before I came along.

They lived in a house on Hale Avenue in the Cincinnati neighborhood of South Avondale. It was a region of big old houses. Along with my Grandmother and Grandfather, the entire family lived in one.

When my mother's sister, Ruth, contracted tuberculosis her two children were sent to Grandma and Grandpa and Mom and Dad. Ruth went to a sanitarium in Chicago. Her husband, Norry, didn't feel capable of taking care of their children, Linda and Joel, by himself. So the kids came to the Hale Avenue house to live.

When they arrived they had tuberculosis as well. It took a year to nurse them back to health, but they eventually healed. They were with the family for five years but when Ruth died Linda and Joel's father took them back. The crisis was over, but the bonding was not.

The experience touched my family deeply. There was great sadness in the death of Mom's sister and the sending away of the kids. But there were also memories of the good times they had together, in this family of four children. I would hear stories about it often. These were legends with the feel of a Golden Age. In comparison I thought my arrival seemed puny and rather out of place.

Barry was the oldest, ten years older than me. Jon was six years older. My parents were old, period. I was a midlife baby. Mom was 39; Dad was 42. I arrived in a terrible storm at 5 a.m. on October sixth, 1952. I was terribly impatient and barely waited for the delivery room. I wanted to arrive and make my presence known.

I've been loudly making my presence known ever since.

I was very much a wanted baby. Mom, who had multiple miscarriages, had been instructed not to get pregnant again. She and Dad decided to risk it anyway. They were hoping for a girl. From what I've been told, everyone was nuts about me at first. Dad called me "Butterball" for my short, round shape and "Rosebud" for my tiny lips.

But there were signs afoot that I was not going to be a sweet little girl. I looked the part – I was immensely cute, if I say so myself. But I didn't sleep. And I cried a lot. This situation led to one of my mother's most oft-told stories. One night she couldn't take it anymore. She called the pediatrician, who was also a friend of the family, and desperately asked him what she could do. "Do what they do in China," he told her. "What's that?" she said. "Bring her to a mountaintop," he replied, "and leave her there."

THE MYSTERY THAT BINDS ME STILL

This certainly was not one of **my** favorite stories. Mom repeated it numerous times until I felt I'd gotten the message. I was a bad girl.

To this day I still have problems sleeping – and when I have one of my restless nights, I *still* feel like I'm a bad girl.

No one knew, of course, that I had attention deficit disorder, anxiety disorder and a panic disorder to boot. I was fidgety and restless all the time. It was classic A.D.D. stuff. I got bored easily and if I was bored I couldn't pay attention for long. Grown-ups kept insisting that being a child, I should take naps. This was forced upon me several times with completely unsuccessful results. I couldn't sleep at night and I certainly couldn't sleep during the day. The worst of it was when I was in kindergarten. We were expected to take naps every day. I tried, but I couldn't hack it. For punishment the teacher made me sit under her desk. I spent a lot of time there, but she had worse things in store. I couldn't figure out how to make my hands do various maneuvers I was expected to do. At home I was having a hellacious time putting on my underpants. Mom worked on it with me, telling me to pretend I was the little engine out of a popular children's book and repeat: "I think I can, I think I can, I think I can." Eventually I figured it out.

But putting on mittens and boots was beyond me. One day I made the great mistake of approaching Mrs. Luis (I think she's probably dead by now; I won't have any problems with libel here) and asking her to help me put on said mittens and boots. The full wrath of this witch descended upon me. She locked me in a dark closet and left me there. What a peach. And I was a bad girl.

There was another kindergarten incident which cemented that thought. We were given some sort of test – one of those standardized how-smart-are-you things – with only pictures, since we didn't know how to read. My family set quite a store about being smart and I was already quite aware of it. So it was bad news when I failed to be able to connect one of the pictures with the word Mrs. Luis said, which was "wreath." Sure enough, there was a picture of a Christmas wreath on the paper, but being Jewish, I had no idea what it was. I got hysterical and my brother Jon was forced to leave his sixth grade class and walk me home.

I must admit that the day Mrs. Luis dropped a milk bottle and got glass shards in her legs and bled – I was glad.

There were other things that I felt set me apart from my family. For one thing, they all looked like each other and I didn't look like any of them. My father called me "the gypsy foundling" and claimed I'd been left on the doorstep. That was another fun family story that got repeated. Also I differed from them physically. They were all tall and beanpole-skinny. I was short and round; cute, but short and round. This shape caused great consternation for Mom and Dad. Although I was not a fat kid they were terrified I was going to turn into one. So no cookie snacks for me and no boxes of candy. Mom got these Russell Stover boxes of candy all the time. Sometimes she'd let me have a piece or two. I longed, however, for a whole box of my own. Finally I was granted that once a year on my birthday. I got a whole box of Turtles, which I loved. However, I was very carefully monitored to make sure I ate only one a day.

At that point my food issues were well underway.

I knew we weren't the family of Beaver Cleaver, but I knew no one was. Still, I'd hear other kids talk about their families having fun together and their siblings being nice now and then. This was not the case for our family, at least it wasn't when I came along. Mom and Dad talked a lot about the things they did with Jon and Barry when they younger, and had energy to do it. This did not make me feel any better about them not doing much with me. If nothing else, Dad strongly bonded with his boys through their playing sports. I was jealous; however, in later years, I heard my brothers' comment that they thought I was spoiled and they resented *me*. Whether it was that or something else, they absolutely hated me. Mom told me that up until I was four they played with me and liked me a lot. I don't know what happened when I was four, but based upon the family experience I'd had so far, I concluded it had to be because I had become a bad girl.

Sibling rivalry and such is common in all families, but the common mythology is that should danger lurk, older siblings will protect the younger ones. Here's an example of how this worked for me. Walking home from school one day I met with some older boys who started pelting me with rocks. Those things *hurt.* I was relieved when I saw Jon come around the corner; I was confident he would prevent them from killing me. Instead, Jon picked up a pile of rocks and commenced throwing them at me too.

I kept to myself as much as possible. Jon was my self-appointed enemy. He had a habit of hitting me quite a bit and they were not playful slaps. They were the real deal. If I tried to hit him back he'd put his hand on my forehead and hold me where all I could do was flail. When I was in sixth grade and sprouted breasts and a period I told him to keep his hands off me because I "was a woman now." Mom and Dad observed this incident and thought it was funny. They all laughed.

Barry basically was just not around. He was off to college when I was pretty young. During the brief years when he and I lived in our house, he limited himself to telling me I was stupid and to some moderate slapping me around. During one semester break from college is when he decided he'd torture me too. On a very rare evening when Mom and Dad were out, he and Jon threw me in the car. They threatened to do terrible things and drove all around. After a few runs around the neighborhood they slowed at a curb and kicked me out. It was completely dark, and I was scared of the dark – which my brothers were fully aware of. They took off and I was utterly paralyzed. About five minutes later they drew up to the curb again. This time they exited the car, grabbed me by my feet and hands and threw me back in. At first I was relieved to hear them say we were heading home. However, upon return they turned me upside down and held me screaming under the running car's exhaust pipe. This was their idea of Fun-In-The-Dark.

My guess is I was in the familiar position in a dysfunctional family – the scapegoat. I was the target for my brothers' anger, disappointment and various moods. For Mom, I was a living confirmation of the "craziness" in the family, and she could both be a martyr because she had a crazy daughter and be relieved, because it took the onus off if I might be crazier than her. For Dad, I had the "precious little girl" role, but outside of that he didn't know what to do with me. Little girls were foreign beings. He was scared of not doing or saying the right things, and of his own lack of understanding. He was scared of me. And I felt it; early on I knew that not only was a very bad girl, but I was a scary person as well.

With that being said, my brothers and I get along now. It's one of my major joys that we've gotten there. We love each other and both of my brothers have gone out of their way to show me how much they care. I'm quite sure that Jon would absolutely defend me now from any rock-throwers; and Barry has let me know he definitely thinks I'm smart. I'm sorry it took so long, but the healing has happened. It is a blessing to finally have sibling acceptance – and love.

Growing up, I had some issues with my father and brothers, specifically. As young as four I was keenly aware that my family was highly pro-male. And I deeply resented it. Dad was the original male chauvinist, often encouraging us all to look out the window and observe the rear end of any attractive female passing by. Playboy magazine was proudly displayed on the coffee table. Once he caught Mom teaching Jon how to sweep the kitchen floor. He grabbed the broom out of Jon's hands and threw it with force against the wall. "No son of mine is doing woman's work!" he yelled. I couldn't figure out what made my gender – and my gender's work - so unacceptable.

It was confusing to me but I imagine it was confusing for my brothers, too. On one hand my dad made it clear how much he appreciated intelligent women, and he generously thought we were all beautiful. "There is no such thing as an ugly woman," he told us. "Just less beautiful ones." He also clearly looked at women as objects made for his enjoyment. It was a rare dinnertime that Dad didn't make excited noises at some female passing by. Mom thought all of this was just fine. She believed it made her more of a woman to have a man who was so much of a man. I concluded that growing up female meant that I was obligated to become a visual treat for all males. It did not make me look forward to womanhood.

Some of my resentment erupted one day at nursery school. It was a Jewish school, so every

THE MYSTERY THAT BINDS ME STILL

Friday we'd celebrate the Sabbath with grape juice, lighting the candles and saying a prayer. That was all fine with me except for one thing - the boys, in keeping with Jewish tradition, got to wear the yarmulkes (skull caps) and the girls didn't. Girls wearing yarmulkes was strictly forbidden. It irritated me for several Sabbaths and one Friday I'd had as much as I could take. I hauled off and hollered and wept and screamed that I wanted to wear a yarmulke too. The teacher tried to speak to me of reason and ancient tradition, but I was not to be placated. To shut me up they finally gave in. I dried my tears and happily plunked a yarmulke on my head.

Maybe I was a young forerunner of the Women's Movement, now that I think of it. There were other incidents, like the day a boy was annoying me so I took a 12x 12 inch wooden block and viciously whopped Ronnie Cohen over the head. It didn't seem to sour him much because later in the year he asked me to marry him. I told him I couldn't answer him right then, because I had to clear it with Mom and Dad.

Mom tried to make me genteel. She tried to teach me how to sew and knit. Mom would use these "sewing cards" which totally bored me and then she'd get mad because I wasn't into it. Clearly, I wasn't happy with being a girl. I couldn't see any profit in it. From the vantage point in my family, it looked like the boys had all the fun.

I had an early desire to be an actor like my dad. I made my debut playing a tree in kindergarten. I went on to take other more complex roles such as "Opie" the disabled boy in the "Pied Piper of Hamelin." I was also a patriot in a play about the American Revolution. I was required to raise my fist in the air and cry out: "No taxation without representation!" and "Down with tyranny!" These were fairly meaty lines but I messed them up. For the life of me I couldn't pronounce "tyranny." It kept coming out "try-annie."

Nonetheless I took on other roles. My favorite was a continually running movie starring me. I pretended the cameras were on me all the time and occasionally stopped what I was doing to pose for a still. This behavior was observed by several of my teachers who puzzled as to the cause of it. No doubt they concluded this was just Another Thing about me that was too eccentric to understand.

In fourth grade I truly blossomed by becoming the founder and president of The Vampire Club. This was a rather exclusive organization involving me and Sandy Berman and Andy Block, two of my friends. We wrote stories about meeting in graveyards on Friday nights, and in art class, Andy was enterprising enough to fashion the Vampire State Building in black paper mache. I wrote to my "Uncle Rod" about it and he answered back with a letter that said he was sorry he was so old, because otherwise he'd send me a couple buckets of blood.

My childhood reflected the quandary I have experienced all of my life. Then as now I am cheerful, spirited; an unsinkable Molly Brown. I am

THE MYSTERY THAT BINDS ME STILL

very enthusiastic, easily excited, and even bombastic. I regard playing as a sort of religion; I love to have fun. On the other hand I am gloomy, pessimistic and sad. Later on when I found out I had bi-polar disorder all this began to make sense. The thing is, I have this disorder, but the illness isn't me. Sandwiched inside there is who I really am. I'd like to think it's a more cheerful me.

Trying to deal with this vague "something wrong" was difficult all around. It was very hard on my folks because they didn't know what to do. Mom gave me my first diagnosis. She said I was "emotionally disturbed." Psychiatry was way, way less of an effective resource than it is today. There were mental hospitals that were still using chains and shackles and shockingly cold baths as "therapy." I was having symptoms galore. For one thing, I peed in my bed every night and did so until I was nineteen years old. I used to wonder how I'd manage to get married; it didn't seem likely I'd find a husband who didn't mind being urinated on.

The whole peeing process was annoying to me altogether. I thought it was an utterly boring waste of time, certainly not something I was willing to interrupt playing to do. I had a lot of wet underpants. To try and prevent this I developed an often used stance. In fact, it's immortalized in my kindergarten photograph. There I am with tightly crossed legs and my hand holding things in to boot. I had a collection of underwear under my bedroom radiator where I put them to dry. Some of them were not peed in; they were merely filled with chocolate pudding or peas I'd put there to avoid having to eat them.

The bladder problem led to a truly hideous experience. The same pediatrician who suggested I be left on a mountain in China decided that I had to get my bladder stretched. To do this I was taken once a month to a doctor's office. Dr. Mullvaney, he was. I'd put him right up there with Mrs. Luis for cruelty. It was years later before I had a name for what was done to me – catheterization - all I knew was that I was put in a little room all alone with this man and he'd shove a tube up my private parts. Than he'd pump liquid up into my bladder, and I still have a vivid memory of the pain. It felt like he was stabbing me with knives in the most humiliating, vulnerable place that he could.

If peeing in the bed hadn't been a symptom of something before, it became one then. I was vulnerable and a little girl, and now I was angry, too. In fact, I was quite literally pissed.

This was illustrated by events on the following Halloween. Mom, an artistic and creative woman who could also sew, made all of our Halloween costumes. They were usually her ideas, too.

This year as in others Jon was assigned to take me on the Halloween appointed rounds. He wasn't happy about being my companion and neither was I. He dealt with it by exacting payment; I was to share half of my candy with him and he had the authority to decide which part of the take I would get.

THE MYSTERY THAT BINDS ME STILL

To his credit, he allowed me at least some of the mini-Hershey bars, the Tootsie Rolls and the packs of M&Ms; but he took most of the good stuff and relegated to me the pennies and the lollipops.

This year Mom got the idea to put us in a costume together. She cut face-sized holes out of sheets. I climbed onto Jon's shoulders while she draped the sheets over us and gave us our masks. Thus we were a giant two-headed ghost.

All went well until my wee bladder had amassed too much to hold, and I peed on Jon's shoulders. He was not pleased. I swear that I did not do it on purpose. But at the same time, I wasn't sorry that it happened.

Uncontrolled peeing was probably my one way to claim my autonomy, to get back at the rest of the family. As in anorexia, they couldn't control my bladder. It was my only individual ownership and a bit of "the hell with you."

The catheterization procedures screwed me up royally. I was only six years old and I didn't have the word for it, but in whatever way I could explain it to myself, I felt raped. From then on I was terrified of men, terrified of sex, terrified at the thought of anything approaching me anywhere near that area again. When I first got my period, I tried to deal with Tampax but seeing that tubular shape coming at me down there totally freaked me out. I was a great disappointment to a lot of boyfriends and men that I dated. There I was, growing up in the sixties, the era of free sex, and I was a frightened and determined virgin.

The treatments were not a success. I still peed in my bed. Until I was ten years old, I wore diapers and rubber pants at night. Only when a therapist suggested to Mom wearing diapers at that age was not a good idea was I then allowed to stop.

If I hadn't already thought I was a bad girl, that bladder procedure settled it. I thought I must have done something horrible to deserve something like this. Not only did I think I was a hideously bad girl, but it started me on the road to hating myself.

At the end of October I was put into the hospital so they could open me up and see what was going on with my bladder. It meant I'd have to stay in the hospital over Halloween! That was too wretched to be borne. But my mom saved the day. In a rare breakout from her depression, she showed her sense of humor, her warmth and her concern. When she wasn't in her dark places Mom had the capacity to be a bit of an eccentric rebel herself. She actually went trick-or-treating for me, going door to door. She wrapped herself in sheets and hung a sign around her neck reading "The Spirit Of Unmade Beds."

At least today I can happily state that I enjoy peeing and I have no problem with it. I particularly enjoy peeing outside, where one can truly appreciate the power and rush of the stream. However, I avoid stinky outhouses. They take away all the joy out of peeing in the clean fresh air.

THE MYSTERY THAT BINDS ME STILL

CHAPTER TWO: NEVER-NEVER-LAND

I grew up on the most magical street in the universe: Glencross Avenue in Cincinnati, Ohio. It was urban and marginally suburban and full of wonders. What made it truly amazing was its location right in the middle of a wood on one side and a busy urban thoroughfare on the other.

The street was absolutely stocked with kids. Big ones, little ones, kids my own age, and sometimes a baby or two. There was always someone to play with; the street rang calls like "Allie Allie in come free" and "Heads up – here comes a car."

There were elderly people too, taking varying roles, some of them Kindly Old Neighbor and some of them the Mean People we usually tried to avoid. Martha was the housekeeper for Mr. Oppenheimer; every Christmas she delivered her gingerbread men to all the neighborhood kids. Mrs. Lena Mayer sat on her porch a lot. If she saw you come by she'd invite you up for a glass of lemonade. The Mean People were spinster and bachelor brothers and sisters who lived in the same house. They kept their blinds and doors shut and hated all human beings that weren't them, but most especially children.

They were fun to tease, though. We'd run up on their lawn and dare ourselves to get as close as we could. They were the only people on the block that wouldn't open their doors to us on Halloween.

At the urban end of the street was Ted's Pharmacy. You'd open the door and see a long marble counter with raised rounded stools you could climb up and twirl on. Behind the counter there were silver shining spigots. From this soda water issued, combining with ice cream to make tall ice cream sodas Ted would sell for 25 cents. For a nickel you could get an ice cream cone, a sundae for a dime. In epicurean awareness Ted was ahead of his time. Snickers and Milky Way bars could not be found in the candy counter. Ted kept them in his freezer where they tasted the best. Another dime could buy you a comic book; Batman, Archie, anything you'd want. Of course, there was medicine there, too.

Down the street from Ted's was Aaron Marmer's grocery store. The Marmers lived in a house that had a buckeye tree, where they let you collect all the buckeyes you wanted. Mr. Marmer liked kids and always provided them with a lollipop when they came in the door. He also gave great barbeques, and we were invited.

Down Glencross Avenue the other way were the houses and the trees. The houses were of the older variety, not Victorian but not modern. The only exception was the house my family lived in when they first moved from Hale Avenue. Mom and Dad built it themselves with the help of Rod Serling and his wife Carol. It had been designed by Benjamin Dunbar who had been a student of Frank Lloyd Wright. The design of the house was pure F.L.W. and kind of stuck out from the rest of the street. We didn't live there long and I barely remember being there. Later the McKenna family bought it, and several years afterward it was nearly consumed by a fire.

The houses were comfortable and welcoming; the trees were too. They were big and beautiful and there were a lot of them. They not only provided us with shade but with toys. Some of them dropped these long cigar-looking things; we played all kinds of games with them. My personal favorite was the sycamores that had large patches of peeling bark. Strips of this bark were perfect to make canoes to float in the gutters or to break into small crunchy pieces and pretend they were chocolate.

At the end of Glencross Avenue there was a forested sanctuary and a mysterious green world. A tarred road broke off of Glencross and descended into the woods, accompanied all the way by wide stone steps. Crabapple trees lined this road, with tiny apples excellent for throwing. Best of all at the end of the road was an arched wooden bridge. Underneath that bridge, a troll lived. Everybody knew that if you didn't run fast enough across it that troll would reach up between the wood, grab you by the ankles, and take you down in the stream to suck your bones. The fact that this had never happened to any of us did not deter us from knowing he was there.

If you braved the troll good stuff awaited you at the end of the bridge. There were three houses there and a circular drive. One was a cottage where elderly people lived but you never saw them in the windows or come out of their house. There were rumors on the street that they ate their dinner as early as *four o'clock* and went to bed at eight! Next to their cottage was an abandoned house with broken windows and a terrible darkness inside. That was the witch's house. The worse thing about it was that it was so black in those window-spaces you couldn't tell whether the witch was looking at you or not.

Then there was the pretty house. It belonged to the Israels'. Mrs. Israel had a breathtaking garden. Some of it hung down a hill sloping into the woods. I thought it was the lost Hanging Gardens of Babylon. She kept Barry employed most of the year, weeding and planting. If the fairies lived anywhere in Glencross Avenue, it would have been there.

A green-skinned boogeyman also lived in those woods but we didn't need to worry about him much because he only came out on Wednesdays. On Wednesdays I made sure to take a different route to school.

Perhaps most compelling was the yawning pit that formed the vast gully in my backyard. Actually it reached across to the Guttman's house next door as well. It was deep and full of junk, old couches and garbage and cast-off food. This made it a perfect environment for rats – huge, monstrous rats the size of cats – that regularly came up out of the gully and frolicked in our backyard. For this reason the backyard was off limits to me. I did all my playing in the front.

Barry told me that the gully was the home of a family of ghosts, headed by a ghost named

THE MYSTERY THAT BINDS ME STILL

Avery. These too came out at night. On Friday nights, they turned themselves into mist. That way they'd come in under the back door and haunt us all night long.

Aggie and Helen Grebber lived on Glencross Avenue. They were not high on my friendship list. For one thing, Aggie broke my Woody Woodpecker whistle five minutes after it arrived, all the way from Battle Creek. Helen's specialty was telling me stuff that would terrify me more than I already was. She told me the devil came in the room if you let the phone ring more than twice. I became very adept at springing for the phone at the first ring. She informed me that witches came out of the toilet when you flushed it. It took me years before I didn't bolt down the stairs, heart hammering, after I flushed. You can be sure I didn't look back. The only thing she told me that I rather enjoyed was that when the sun is out and rain is falling, it means the devil is getting married. That image has fascinated me ever since.

Mom didn't cotton to Helen's stories. After all, she was the one who sat with me when I couldn't sleep or was awakened when I had nightmares, which happened often. Mom was the one who took all the fallout from my fears. She concluded that both of us had had enough. One day she marched down to the Grebber's house, walked in the door without knocking, and spanked Helen then and there, right in front of her parents. It was unbelievable arrogance, but Mom could be as righteous as Dad. When she got mad enough she was convinced she was doing the right thing and God help anyone who got in her way.

Glencross Avenue had 50% Jewish and 50% Catholic. This also added to my spiritual confusion. We all got along as far as religion was concerned although I do recall an incident which unfortunately ended in one camp calling "Jewish-Schmuish!" and another "Catholic-Smatholic!" Hearing this, Dad charged over to the door and let us know that we would be tolerant or he would break our heads.

One thing we all enjoyed playing was church. Both Debbie Guttmann (my next door neighbor and best friend) and I were fascinated with the rituals of Catholicism. The Grebber kids had a rather gruesome perspective on their religion. I never heard them talk about anything comforting such as the love of the Virgin Mary or the ministering of Christ, but they were fond of describing, in lurid detail, his wounds. If Debbie or I had any sort of accident that would cause us to cry we were told to hush and consider the bravery of Jesus on the cross. We were told about the fires of Hell that awaited us, which was news to me because Jews generally don't believe in a physical Hell. However, Helen and Aggie swore to it and I swore that I was going there, too.

To play church, Helen and Aggie lined up folding chairs in the basement. They mumbled words that they said were prayers and then came to each of us with a little ball of Wonder bread. I was traumatized by Helen who told me "Put this in your mouth, but don't swallow it. It's Jesus."

THE MYSTERY THAT BINDS ME STILL

I was nervous, and gulped. To my horror I realized I had swallowed the bread. I took off crying and ran home, bursting into the kitchen to Mom. "Help me!" I cried. "I've swallowed Jesus!"

As I recall, my mother was just not prepared to deal with this at all.

All of the kids, young and old, played Pickle and Dodge Ball, Stickball and War, switching when it was twilight to Ghost-In-The-Graveyard and our all-time favorite, Hide-And-Go-Seek. At eight o'clock the streetlights came on and we had to stop. Most nights we'd gather on Debbie Guttman's porch, and I'd tell stories.

Storytelling came naturally to me. Everyone in my family told stories. We rarely ever did any activity as a family but when we gathered at the dinner table we each in turn told about our day. Dad loved to tell stories from his life. Our favorite, and Mom's least favorite, was the time he helped you-know-who with his horse and wagon and the horse pooped on Dad's head. I was fascinated with acting and speech making, writing stories and telling them. Dad encouraged me completely. I told my stories at camp and school as well as in the neighborhood.

I made my daydreaming an art. If I was playing in a water sprinkler, I was a water sprite. In the back of North Avondale School was a copse of trees and a large rock. I used to sit on the rock and weave tales about how I was really a princess but I was held captive in a castle and made to work as a scullery maid. Subconsciously it was a tale about my position in the family. I had no idea then that this story would be a metaphor for my life, which I spent hiding and pretending and knowing I was more than I appeared – but being terrified that if I showed who I was no one would like it.

I loved my princess daydreams. They telegraphed to me that I was special. At a time when I hated myself they provided my only feelings of self-love. In my "dreamtime" little of what was truly happening concerned me. I wasn't there. I made my own worlds. For me, imagination was not just storytelling - it was a spiritual, sacred thing that kept me alive.

Sometimes the only way I could hold on to being a princess was to hide. When I didn't know someone or when I was in large crowds or at a social event, I'd just shut up. If I said anything I was convinced it was stupid and everyone could see the awkward "scullery maid" that I was. The only way I could avoid this behavior was by showing off. If I was entertaining or in the spotlight, I was fine. I learned early on that being bombastic gave me safety. Otherwise, I was timid, even shy.

Being a princess took on different themes. Most often, as in masquerading as a scullery maid, I was trying not to reveal that I was crazy and scary and inappropriate, all the things I believed I was. Except when I was magical. Except when I was a princess.

I was in my late thirties when I discovered I was supposed to have been given a Hebrew name when I was born. Both of my brothers had their *bris,* the ceremony for the removal of the foreskin. The naming ceremony was the girls' version of being welcomed into the world. I asked my rabbi: "What is the Hebrew name for 'princess?"

"Sara," he said. He pronounced it in the Hebrew way, "SAR-AH. I'll do a naming ceremony for you."

Thus I was reborn. I bought a pretty dress and lit the candles, made a speech and became a real "princess." Sar-ah Bat Yisrael, princess, daughter of Israel.

Several years ago I decided I could claim my "princessness" in other ways if I wanted to, so from time to time I referred to myself as "Princess Mickie of York." It amuses others and delights me. Sometimes you have to take your dreams into your own hands.

My vivid imagination also fed my fears. I had a lot of them, along with rituals and warding-off-evil habits. I kept my fingers permanently crossed for months, hoping it would bring me luck. I dug chunks out of my hair, and had to touch the walls in a particular way whenever I entered a room. I never looked at a mirror in the dark because I knew a monster would be there instead of my face. Looking back, I believe that was the beginning of incipient O.C.D., my first taste of rituals and compulsive behavior.

Being the youngest I was the first upstairs to bed. I was scared of the dark and of being alone. I was terrified to be away from the comfort of people and the familiar blare of the television. I had to sleep facing the wall because some hideous being might be standing in the doorway, or I might see Marley's ghost forming on my closet door. To stay on my side I had to hold my body so stiffly it was extremely uncomfortable which added to my reluctance to go to bed. When Barry went to college Mom put me in his room, thinking that would eliminate my fears. His room had a long mirror on the door and that made everything worse; I knew that if I looked at it something indescribable would be looking back at me. My solution to this was to ignore it as best I could, but it didn't work. I did a lot of calling Mom up from downstairs. After she refused to do it anymore I read by a flashlight until everyone else came up to bed.

I know now I had panic and anxiety disorder. But nobody knew that back then. As a child I was already having symptoms of these disorders. One of them was that I always felt like I had a lump in my throat. I recall a doctor's visit about that one, and my mother's doubt that I was telling the truth. The intensity of my fears was known at home and obvious at times elsewhere. I don't know what people concluded, although I was aware that some of them, including my brothers, viewed me with contempt. All I knew was that I was in a constant state of fear. I woke up scared, I went to bed scared. Once I got to sleep I had nightmares. (I still do, every night.) If Mom wouldn't let me get into bed with her I'd lay a blanket next to her bed and sleep there.

THE MYSTERY THAT BINDS ME STILL

When I was four two big things happened. We moved across the street to a bigger house and Grandpa died. I have been told that Grandpa and I were very close although I barely remember him. But the memories I have are sharp, going back to when I was two and three years old. So he must have been important to me.

Mom said he adored me. That must have felt good as I didn't feel welcome with anyone else in the family. In my earliest years Mom appeared angry, Dad seemed scary, my grandmother got mad at me for spending so much time in the bathroom – and of course my brothers didn't care for me at all.

Unfortunately my sharpest memory of being with him is getting mad because he chose to watch Arthur Godfrey on television when I wanted to see "Uncle Al." It strikes me as significant that I remember this time when I got angry at someone, rather than a family member being mad at me. I must have felt comfortable with him or I wouldn't have done that. Anyone else in the house wouldn't have tolerated it.

I dimly recall seeing him in bed once and being told he had a cold. I never saw him after that. Mom kept me out of his room. On the day he died of cancer I didn't know it. But I must have suspected something, because I clearly recall being sent to spend the day with my cousin. I remember being driven to Dayton and then back home when it was dark and the moon was up. "The moon is following us," I told them, "The moon is following us" repeating it several hundred more times.

Grandpa had been there and then he wasn't and no one ever told me where he went. Mom thought she had spared me, thinking that if I wasn't allowed to see him I'd forget he was there. It didn't work. This incident added greatly to what I would experience later in panic episodes. I also developed a sense of abandonment. For the rest of my life I was afraid that people I cared about would disappear, not show up when they said they would or not show up at all. When someone was late and I didn't know where they were or what had happened to them I would be seized with paralyzing fear. I couldn't move or breathe until they showed up or called. I'd make anxious phone calls to their friends or family or places of work, or I'd call a friend to help me not feel alone until the one I was waiting for walked in the door. I was easily certain someone I loved was dead – or didn't love me anymore or worse, was simply gone and I did not know where or why. Like Grandpa.

Some of my fears I have picked up from Mom who had more than enough foreboding to spare. Her fears led to a lot of things I didn't know at that time, even the reason we lived on Glencross Avenue. Mom was terrified to leave the house. If she had to go she couldn't go far; one block formed her region of safety. Glencross had a drug and grocery store at the corner of the road - this was her requirement. Up until my teens I was her official accompaniment to either of these places. I thought she was taking me with her when we went shopping – I didn't know until much later that I was taking her. I was also appointed to make sure she was never alone. Barry and Jon escaped these duties; in fact, I'm not sure they even knew of Mom's demands or how much they involved me.

We did not have a car because Mom was afraid to drive. I don't know why Dad wouldn't either, but we weren't a mobile family. We didn't have the kind of bonds other families may have had that I heard about, who went on vacations, took Sunday drives or went out to eat. We never went out to eat; that was Dad's edict. During his youthful wanderings he had been poor and close to starving. "For one whole month I ate nothing but apple butter," he told us. He never allowed a jar of apple butter in his presence again.

We were not allowed to go on picnics or to restaurants. Dad said he had suffered enough and wanted only homemade food. Whether this made Mom suffer did not seem to occur to him. Picnics were on the forbidden list because we would have to contend with bugs. "I spent enough of my life fighting for my food," Dad would growl. "I'm never doing it again."

Being together at dinner served as our bond and it centered on food and talk. To this day I have a fondness and a penchant for both.

For a while Mom valiantly tried to drive. I remember us having some sort of blue Chevrolet. After a year, way too shaken to continue, she called it quits. Because she couldn't bear to be without my father he quit his job as a foreman in an upholstery shop downtown and set up his own shop in our basement. Not only was starting his own business dicey, but he was also taking a chance with the law. Businesses were not allowed in a residential district such as Glencross was.

Mom and Dad almost never went out; I can probably count the number of times they did on one hand. Babysitters were an unknown breed for me. The few times my parents left the house without me I was put in the care of my brothers, never a good idea. When Mom found out what they did to me while she was gone she was even less compelled to go out.

Consequently I was rarely alone. Later when I moved into my first apartment I could never settle in to feeling it was okay to be by myself. I was nervous and ill at ease all the time. I felt unnatural and all but held my breath until I saw other human being again.

On the occasions that Mom, Dad or I had a doctor's or dentist's appointment, we'd go together, taking a bus or a cab. Sometimes Dad would treat us an ice cream or a movie. Just once Dad went downtown without her. Mom wouldn't let me go outside. She made me stay in the living room with her until Dad came home so she wouldn't have to be alone. I remember wanting to go outside and play and Mom being bitter because I wasn't loyal enough to her to want to stay by her side. I was all of seven years old.

When Jon turned 17 they helped him buy a car and he had to ferry us around. This did not make him happy, but it made it possible for me to visit friends outside of my immediate neighborhood. I also got to do nifty things, like take oil painting lessons, because a friend's parents were willing to drive me there. Mom wanted me to take the lessons because she was an excellent artist. She was hoping I'd end up liking to paint, which I did.

Painting was, and still is, a fascination for me. I love anything that allows me to create what wasn't there before. Doing so with colors that become shape and dimension is magic. Today I enjoy painting murals, especially on garage doors. It gives individuality to the homeowner and a vast canvas for me. I've painted eclectic gardens, landscapes, scenes from "The Wizard of Oz," battleships and mermaids under the sea. It's immensely fun and gives me my happiest connection to Mom.

Other fun activities came from my Grandma, who would have me stay at her house for ten days at a time. She was nasty to me while Grandpa was still alive; apparently she didn't care for him and she got nicer after he died. She would spoil me completely. We'd walk to the corner for ice cream, or she'd make me hot pineapple juice with a cinnamon stick for a straw. When Cincy schools closed for "Zoo Day" it was Grandma who would take me every year. She didn't have a car either but we'd travel by bus or cab. She gave me my first taste of culture by taking me to the opera. Cincinnati had a very unusual opera house then – it was located in the Cincinnati Zoo. One could hear peacocks screeching and lions roaring over the arias. I liked "Carmen," which was pretty lively. But "Madame Butterfly" and such made me fidgety and bored. As a whole, Grandma's operatic sojourns with me did not take hold.

I looked upon my grandmother as rather magical, too. She was beautiful and she had snow white hair. She listened to music all day, baked wonderful things, and gardened. I loved watching her big white moonflowers that visibly opened at dusk. When I think of her, that's the image I get: the Moonflower Lady, flowering in the night.

Grandma's indulgence was wonderful stuff. My mother was a maniac about the basic food groups. People eating doughnuts for breakfast or more than one starch at a time just appalled her to no end. But Grandma let me eat whatever I liked. I remember one glorious Saturday downtown when she took me to a buffet. She let me select an unheard of meal of macaroni, cornbread, coconut pie and chocolate cake. I haven't forgotten it, to this day.

The other great joy in my life was camp. Camp Cincio-Cinciette was an all-gender Jewish day camp in a Cincinnati park called Winton Woods. Jon and Barry were counselors and I was a camper. All three of us loved it, a rare thing we had in common. Every summer I couldn't wait to go. The camp bus picked us up for a full day of activities including twirling, fencing, and learning Hebrew dances. Barry and I took to the dancing, which became a bond for the two of us. We also loved the camp songs. I don't know how many there were but it seemed like there were a zillion of them. I remember some of them vividly: Johnny Verbeck who ground up dogs and cats in his machine; the moonshine song, Mountain Dew, the intolerably loud John Jacob Jingleheimer Schmidt and most especially, Johnny Appleseed and The Boogie-Woogie Three Bears Song, two songs I use in my storytelling performances today. Sprinkled throughout we learned Hebrew songs too, doing hand movements to David Melech Yisrael, relishing the whizzing sounds in Zum Gali, Gali, tearing it up in a wild Hava Nagila. My love of the songs and dances became another hook that drew me occasionally into Judaism.

Our house had two stories with the bathroom on the second floor. Dad had a primitive kind of john in the basement where he would go when he was working. Once on the main floor, if he needed to go to the bathroom he climbed the stairs. A childhood bout with Scarlet Fever left him with an enlarged heart. Mom was quite frantic about it, fearing he'd have a heart attack. So she asked me to release him from the duty of coming to the second floor to tell me goodnight. This made no sense to me at all, given that he had to climb those self-same stairs to go to the bathroom or to go to bed. Why it was coming to me what was going to kill him? This was the beginning of my awareness of several things, all of which grew in intensity later on. According to Mom, Dad was always dying; I was the one who was going to kill him, and she didn't want me to have too much intimacy with him as she felt in competition. Later on, when they moved to California, she wrote me a letter accusing me of trying to take him away from her. "Don't you know it's no use - he's mine." she wrote. I literally threw up.

I was tight with my next-door buddy, Debbie Guttman. I'd tell stories; she'd draw pictures for them. Occasionally she'd forsake me for Jill Anderson. She and her brother Sandy were sort of the thugs in the neighborhood. We certainly didn't all get along, nor were we always loyal friends, but we were available to each other, and that counted a lot. The kids from camp and the neighborhood were my world. I needed them to escape from my parents who told me they were "too old" to play with me and it was a shame I wasn't around when they were young enough to play with Barry and Jon. I needed them to escape Mom's sharp criticism and her fears, the harshness of my brothers and the loneliness I felt in that quiet house, where my brothers were out playing sports and my parents were reading or watching TV. Most of all, I needed them to escape my inner demons, the fears that engulfed me along with the sense there was something wrong.

Glencross Avenue and its denizens filled my emptiness and kept my head above water. When I was nine we moved to Bond Hill and it all came crashing down.

THE MYSTERY THAT BINDS ME STILL

CHAPTER THREE: BOY'S GYM SHOES

Glencross Avenue was in North Avondale. North Avondale was a neighborhood known for its open-minded people, their tolerance, and their sense of fun. Even North Avondale Elementary School was considered "experimental," with teachers and teaching way out of the box.

At school teachers approved my ability of writing and storytelling. If what I wrote was unusual they accepted it, even liked it all the more. Except for the strictness of some of the teachers there and of course, the usual rules, I remember North Avondale School as kind of a loose, happy place. The principal, Mrs. Reske, had a sense of humor. I remember the sign she put up on the faculty lunchroom door: "Reske's Hideaway," it read.

The move to Bond Hill was truly a traumatic experience. Mom and Dad had done it because they were always afraid Dad would be caught for running a business in a residential neighborhood. The house at 1221 California Avenue was in a district zoned for business. Per requirement, the house was less than a block from a grocery store. Dad set up shop in the basement there, and I began a lonely life of living next door to a hardware store and a bar, with nary a kid in sight.

The lack of kids wasn't the only problem. Bond Hill seemed to be the polar opposite of North Avondale – I found it to be much more conservative and traditional, and when I entered

Bond Hill Elementary School I was to find that the kids there had some very different ideas of what constituted fun.

However there were good things that came out of it. I met Sue, a much older teen down the street who had radical ways and ideas. She embodied all of the sixties ideals. I was already influenced by Barry's activities breaking up segregation for the Congress of Racial Equality (C.O.R.E.) and his going to Antioch College, which was as experimental as a college could be. When Sue came along I was already ripe; so as a nine year old radical, I was ready to be launched.

I was introduced to Ted and Martha's Variety Store up the street. This became a haven for me. Within the first lonely week Mom gave me a quarter and sent me there to buy some amusement for myself. I wandered among the aisles, star struck at all the wealth of treasure there: candy bars, model cars, scotch tape, red rubber balls. I was nuts about scotch tape, so that was my first choice. On the next visit I chose a red rubber ball.

I loved both tape and balls for the same reason; they presented possibilities. All sorts of things might be done with them. I still like anything that can be made into something that wasn't originally there. I think of it as re-creating the universe. Writing qualifies as that, too. Today I'm more of a fan of colored duct tape than scotch tape and I have added on a new love, extension cords – the longer the better, and preferably colored blue or even pink.

THE MYSTERY THAT BINDS ME STILL

It turned out that Kotter's hardware store next door served me well. I took my red rubber ball into the driveway, bounced it, and then batted it against Kotter's wall. I did this for countless hours after school and during summer days. The whole time I was not only becoming immensely dexterous, I was weaving tales in my head. These stories were about a whole dynasty that played this game (whatever it was), their joys and their tragedies. My stories were like soap operas, on a pre-adolescent scale.

The Kotters were the first anti-Semites I met. They hated Jews and knew we were Jewish. However, they were okay with us and said so. "You're white Jews," they said, whatever that meant. It was the same logic I found in all my encounters with Jew-haters. Bond Hill harbored quite a few.

Jon, who now lived in the attic, amused himself by removing a foot of soil off the top of our entire backyard. This revealed hundreds of tiny oyster-like shells. They fascinated me. It was my first foray into archeology and science. It turned out Bond Hill had once been part of a vast lake, or most certainly in ancient times, the ocean. While Jon dug, I would occasionally keep him company in the manner that allowed me to amuse myself as well. This was whirling about and declaring in a falsetto voice: "I am the merry sprite of spring; I spread my joy over everything!" For some reason this made Jon laugh. Score one for my first positive experience with my brother.

On my first day of school I walked into the playground in my usual way, with a hearty walk and pumping arms. To my surprise a girl blocked me and stood in my way. She imitated me and laughed, pointed me out to kids all over the place. It was not a good start.

This girl (unfortunately, here I *do* fear libel, so I'll change her name) was Shirley Ann Gretzman. She was, for reasons unclear to me then and equally unclear to me now, the most popular girl in school. She decided right away to hate my guts.

She was very good at this. Never believe that a ten year old girl cannot be a vicious, full-fledged bitch because I fully attest she can.

It wasn't long before Ms. Gretzman began to follow me about, declaring in her unattractive nasal voice: "Oh, you're SO queer!" Actually, it came out more like this: "Oh, you're soooo queheere!" The other kids picked this up and soon they were all addressing me in this same manner: "Oh, you're SO queer!"

If by this phrase they meant to indicate I did not fit in, they were correct. At ten, I was still interested in playing softball and Hide-and-go-Seek. These kids were playing spin-the-bottle, attending ballroom dance classes and going on dates.

The crowning incident occurred around Gym Day. On this appointed Day – and *only* this appointed Day, were we allowed to wear our sneakers to class. Mom took me to the shoe store to buy my sneakers. She immediately headed to the girls' shoes which featured delicate pink Keds lined with little pink lace. I stood my ground. I was NOT going to wear girls' gym shoes, I told her, and that was that. I had never created such a rebellion. Mom was beside herself. She threatened me with everything from grounding to no dinner but I held firm. She had no choice. I came away from the store with what I dearly wanted – *boy's* gym shoes like my brothers,' wide, white and rubbery with big thick laces. Not a touch of pink.

I was walking down the hall on Gym Day, wearing my happy new gym shoes, when Shirley Ann was coming up the other way. She looked at my feet. She stopped, and put her hands on her hips. She expelled her breath on the air. "Why," she began, "Why –"she sputtered, smacking then pursing her lips – "WHY are you wearing – boy's – GYM SHOES?????"

I answered her with the first thing that came to my mind. "Well, I'm not really a girl," I said. "I used to be a boy but a wicked witch put a spell on me and put me in the shape I am now. But my feet know the difference."

It was all over school in an hour. "Mickie Singer is a liar." I was terribly hurt. It was the first time anyone had ever mistaken one of my stories for a lie.

There were other reasons why I didn't fit in. I was curious. I raised my hand and asked questions. Apparently, this just wasn't *done*. When I was assigned to write a Thanksgiving story I wrote about an ear of corn that didn't want to be eaten so he jumped off the table and ran away. My teacher told me I had written worthless nonsense and gave me an F.

If I went to someone's house and I was offered something to eat, I generally took it and said thank you. My parents didn't consider that wrong. But there seemed to be a whole different standard for the children of Bond Hill. According to them not only was I "queer," I was rude.

It was an adjustment for all of us, moving from free-thinking North Avondale to the more austere Bond Hill. At least we kept our sense of humor. One Saturday morning Mom called loudly from the bedroom, "Mickie, wake up! It's eight o'clock! You're going to be late for school!"

Heart hammering, I shot out of bed. Then it hit me. I crawled back into bed and lay down. Mom yelled again: "MICKIE!!"

"Mo," I yelled back, "It's Saturday."

"Oh," you're right," she said, and all was quiet again.

Except for Dad, who sometimes had a delayed reaction. He sat up in bed and in a most aggrieved tone said "What was that yelling all about?"

I shouted back, "It's Saturday!"

"I *know* it, GODDAMIT!" he shouted in reply.

The Bond Hill experience sunk my already wavering self-esteem. As I would remark to people later, I never had a problem with low self-esteem. I had NO self-esteem.

THE MYSTERY THAT BINDS ME STILL

Except for the support of Sue and later other friends, I thought of myself as unacceptable and inappropriate – and crazy to boot. At times I hated myself so intensely I went into a rage, wishing I could tear away my skin and be gone. Sometimes I had thoughts of suicide.

This "not fitting in" thing seemed to extend beyond Bond Hill. Since I didn't get around much other than downtown and in the neighborhood, I thought of the outer world as a mysterious and extraordinary place. This especially applied to Nature, which I saw little of. Once I was on a camping trip with some other kids and my socks got wet so I borrowed a pair from one of the girls. I went off by myself to take a walk along a creek. I felt like I was in wonderland, watching the water swirl around the rocks and listening to the rushing of the stream. On the bank, I suddenly came upon a dead fish. Now *this* was an amazing find, I thought, worthy of being shared with others. So I took off one of the socks I was wearing and wrapped the dead fish in it. Then I hurried back to camp. "Look everybody!" I yelled. "Look what I found!" I unrolled the sock and revealed the lifeless fish.

To my astonishment, not only were they not pleased with my offering, they actually said "Euueeeew" and the girl who owned the sock wailed "No! No! That was my sock!"

I remember meeting with my appointed Big Sister with the other little sisters a week before we were to enter 7th grade. A very earnest and well-meaning girl, she asked each of us to describe ourselves. The other three girls reported generally on their families, pets and sports of choice. When it was my turn I quoted straight out of "Peter Pan" – "I am youth, I am joy," I said. "Ah, one of *those,*" my Big Sister replied. I could tell by her tone I'd said something wrong. The other girls eyed me as if I were extremely weird.

Apparently I was still so queer.

In sixth grade my parents sent me to my first psychiatrist. Mom had wanted to send me for several years, but Dad wouldn't hear of it. No daughter of *his* – yadda yadda yadda. Later they told me that what changed his mind was when I announced to them in absolute earnest that I had just had a conversation with my dead Aunt Ruth. This was supposed to have occurred when Aunt Ruth was on the roof. I was rather obsessed with her; I slept with a quilt she had made and Mom had given me her name for my middle one. The funny thing about it was that I have no memory of the conversation – and no memory of telling them I had it. If I had to guess I'd bet I actually had the conversation with her. Aunt Ruth probably told me to report it to my parents so Dad would finally let me see a shrink.

I don't remember much about this therapy but I doubt it did much good. The doctor was a nice man but this was when psychiatry was pre-knowledge about so many things. I would track in and out of many therapists' offices over the years and no one knew what to do with me, least of all myself.

THE MYSTERY THAT BINDS ME STILL

CHAPTER FOUR: I WAS A TEENAGE WEREWOLF

When I was eleven I turned into a walking freak show. I was always small for my age. I reached four feet 10 and a half inches, and stopped growing forever. Vertically, that is. My chest, on the other hand, thrust out like the peaks of the Matterhorn.

Physically I resembled the Goodman women on my mother's side. My grandmother and all my great aunts were short, broad-shouldered, hefty, and had big boobs. My mother was well endowed too. But I beat 'em all.

Some of this came from the encouragement of candy purchased daily at the candy store across from Bond Hill School. At that point my parents' fears came true. I started to get a trifle pudgy. But the most distinctive thing about me was my titanic chest.

I imagine this short kid with massive breasts must have been quite a sight. All I knew was everywhere I went people stared at me and I didn't know why. This added to my paranoia about being inappropriate, and also convinced me that I was truly losing it. For that reason I never said anything about it to my parents. Finally I got my courage up and told Mom and Dad people were looking at me. The next time we went on a trip downtown Dad deliberately walked behind me and took notice of the faces of folks passing by. I was right, he said. Everyone stared. Then he told me why.

Mickie R. Singer

His advice was "if you've got it, flaunt it."

I didn't mind having a large chest. It was part of my body, part of me, and that had to be okay. I was used of being considered unusual anyway. It was some of the attention I got that I minded a great deal.

When I got old enough to go out by myself I had to take a bus. Sometimes I had to take multiple buses involving several transfers and several bus stops. As a result I was often subject to comments made as cars went by or pulled to the curb. These were sometimes insults, sometimes threats, always intrusive and shaming.

"Give me some of that sugar," I'd hear, or "You're like a chimney – stacked." "It takes two hands to handle a whopper," one would say. There were various assortments of "Oh baby," whistles and sometimes a downright menacing. "Come 'ere, sweet thing. I'm gonna give it to you. Then you'll know what it's like with a real man."

Once when I was walking home from school a man began to walk past me then shot out his hand. Roughly he cupped my breast, then removed his hand with such force that it broke my necklace. I felt like less than nothing, powerless, just standing there with a broken necklace on the ground.

As a result of my bladder treatments I was already scared of men. These incidents didn't help. Neither did my mother's views on the subject. When I was 14 she gave me her Talk about dating. "You should know that *every single boy* you go out with will try to get in your pants,"

64

she told me. "Just be prepared. Always carry some money with you so that if you need to you can come home in a cab."

As far as I was concerned, dating sounded like a wrestling match. I pledged to have none of it and didn't until college. Even then I found it artificial and tense. I was lucky that in the sixties "dating" per se was considered not cool by the folks I hung around with. Within the hanging around process I had occasional romantic dalliances, which kept me happy to some extent – but not very. Most of my crowd paired off and I desperately wanted a genuine boyfriend.

I didn't like my bus stop experiences. But they gave me one advantage: a determinedly protective edge. In my teens I was stupid enough to hitchhike. One day the inevitable occurred. I was picked up by a guy who leaned over, muttering "I think I'll just close the window," and in so doing rubbed his hands against my chest. My reaction and response were immediate. We were going around the corner at 30 miles an hour but I didn't care. I threw myself out of the car.

He yelled some expletives but traveled on. I picked myself up off the ground, a little bruised, but reassured to know that when I needed to I'd take care of myself.

On another occasion I was waiting at a bus stop downtown around 11 p.m. with a female friend. A cab pulled up at the corner stuffed with the driver and five other men. They were American Legionnaires, in town for a convention, and high on a lot more than life. They started heckling us; all the same dumb stuff. "Come here, honey," cried one of them. "I'm coming, honey," I answered, concealing a 32 ounce cup of sticky orange drink behind my back. It was a hot summer night; all the windows were open. When I got close enough I tossed the orange drink through the windows, taking great care that each Legionnaire got his fair share.

The cab rounded the corner and screeched to a dead stop. I could hear them shouting to the driver: "Stop the cab! We're gonna kill the bitch." I was fired up. I raised my fists and went into a fighter's stance, all four feet ten of me, and yelled back: "I'm ready for you! Come on!"

They drove off.

It was ludicrous behavior, but I was sixteen. And mad.

I was a teenager during the sixties, which had started early for me. I belonged to a Labor Zionist group called Habonim. It was an organization dedicated to taking action as a Jew, which in Zionism meant going to Israel and living there. In Habonim, it meant living at a socialist *kibbutz.* In America you would train for the day you would go there (make *aliyah).*

For the first couple of years I loved it. With its teaching of Hebrew language, songs and dances, Habonim gave me a clear identity. Better yet, it was based on nationalist Judaism, not religious Judaism, which fit me just fine. My religious education was sorely wanting, limited to Grandma making Rosh Hashonah dinner and taking me to Temple a couple of times. When all

THE MYSTERY THAT BINDS ME STILL

the many movements of the sixties took hold, most of the people in Habonim went right along. Unfortunately, this also included the usage of drugs.

My first experience of such activities took place in 7th grade when I was a sleepover hostess for a fellow girl in Habonim. The purpose was so she could hide from her parents and take morning glory seeds. The buzz was the seeds gave the same effect as LSD, and unlike later claims of intoxicants in banana peels, it worked. She was quite transported, and I thought myself extremely cool.

That episode was the first of many in which I was always in the midst of other people taking drugs. I quickly came to hate it; once again I was different, left out. But I couldn't bring myself to "smoke grass," "drop acid," or do any of these myriad types of activities my friends did. I was plain scared.

I think I sensed I was already way out of control, just being me; I didn't need anything to make me more so. But the people who accepted and liked me, and who I liked in turn, did dope. Period. For years I participated in the same weekend ritual. We'd get together in a circle and pass a joint. I would pass it by. Everybody else would get stoned and act like assholes.

This wasn't too much fun for me so I decided to do something about it. To avoid having my friends' think of me as not one of them, I took to taking the joint when it came along. A couple of years ago Bill Clinton announced he'd tried pot but never inhaled. The whole country laughed at him. Not me. I believed him, because I did the same thing.

I'd make a viable production out of putting the joint in my mouth, making sucking noises, and looking like I was blowing out. Then I'd pass it on to the next one.

After a while that didn't do it either. I resolved to finally try the stuff; I just couldn't bring myself to decide when. My friend Harold took care of the matter for me. When I was at his house he produced a bong and a quantity of hashish. "You're getting stoned," he announced, and showed me how to work the pipe. In the language of the vernacular, I got wasted.

I hated that, too. I got the munchies and the gigglies and all that, but I also got a heavy dose of paranoia. I could tell feeling stoned could be pleasurable, but I spent most of the time trying not to feel it. As I'd suspected, I couldn't stand the feeling of not being in control.

I went back to being honest and anti-drug. Not being under the influence I had the vantage point to see how dope changed my friends. Some of them weren't too happy. Take Denny, for instance. He had dropped acid and was on the edge of a bad trip. He told Michele to please not open her mouth because her teeth were terrifying him. Steve fell on a field of glass and had to be taken to the emergency room. Debby, Joanie and all the rest who smoked their joints "shit on" people and turned uncharacteristically mean. Fred fried his brains to the point he kept the lights on so nothing he had seen on his "trips" could get him in the dark. Years later, when I was no longer in the group, Tom put a gun to his head.

At the time I thought the whole drug taking thing was just dumb. And so was I. For one thing, I actually believed that if our group ever got "busted" I'd be safe because everyone would explain to the cops that I didn't do drugs. I was right there at times when someone was dealing heroin or cocaine. I thought I was surrounded by some kind of bubble, and in a way I was. I was capable of being way too streetwise and entirely naïve – all at the same time. I had selective seeing and selective hearing. If I didn't want to recognize it, it wasn't there. At times this "who, me?' attitude got me into such trouble it was amazing I got out of it.

Case in point: I'm wandering down the street of Mt. Adams, one of the most "hip" Cincinnati neighborhoods. It clung to a hill and gave breathtaking views of the city. A lot of artists lived there. All you had to do to be considered hip was to walk down a Mt. Adams street. If you lived there, you were beyond hip, you were groovy.

So I made it my business to walk down the Mt. Adams streets. That day I said 'hi' to a good looking guy I barely knew. Suddenly he started hitting on me. But I didn't realize it because I was in my bubble. Besides, I could never recognize anyone was flirting with me because I never believed I was worth flirting with. But he was laying it on thick, and it got through to me that *something* was going on.

His interest in me was high flattery. Not only was he known to be hip among the people who hung around Mt. Adams, he actually *lived* there. In fact, he invited me to his apartment. And I went, sheep to the slaughter, never suspecting a thing.

As soon as we got inside his apartment door, he began in earnest to try to convince me to screw him. "I've always loved you," he said.

I just laughed. "I hardly think that's possible since you don't even know my name!"

Thus it continued, him laying it on, me laughing it off until he pitched his strongest ball. "But you must make love to me," he begged, "I'm going away tomorrow and I'll never see you again."

"Bon voyage!" I told him airily. I didn't understand why he looked so pissed off when I called a cab and left.

I suppose I was in my bubble when I went to see the movie "Monterey Pop" with a group of my friends. We were excited about seeing it. Pre-Woodstock, "Monterey Pop" was a film of one of the first rock festivals. Janis Joplin was in it, as an up and coming singer. I would watch that little woman grind her feet to the floor and wail and I was gone. Nobody, before or since, could deliver a song in her transcendent style.

Before the film we watched a "short." Back then instead of watching previews we'd watch a short film or cartoon. On this occasion it was a short about Texas. As I watched I saw a man lift up a horse's foot and hammer on a horseshoe. I was struck dumbfounded by utter revelation. I leapt to my feet and cried out: "My God! My God! Horseshoes are shoes for *horses*!!!"

My friends were embarrassed and the audience roared, but I didn't know. I was a city girl who rode around on a bus. I thought horseshoes were a game, or something you nailed up above a door for luck.

Dad was still my hero, especially the way he sometimes stood between me and Mom. Mom hid her illness in the outside world. It was the same thing I would do as well. Everyone who knew her outside of the family thought of her as good-humored, good-hearted and warm. The thing is she *was* all those things. She adored Dad and would never think of messing with her sons, but her sadness had to go somewhere. I was the target.

As a kid, she gave to me her disapproval and disappointment. At four I confided to her that I wanted to be a TV star. I loved to sing, I loved to dance and I loved to act. I dreamed of doing something great.

She nipped that one in the bud. "You're not a good enough singer or dancer or actor and you never will be," she informed me. "You'd better give up that dream."

I was so crushed I cried all night long.

She often took a very snide tone. I remember asking her the definition of a word that I couldn't figure out. It was "gentlewoman," a term I had read in a book. I knew what a gentleman was, but I asked Mom what was a "gentlewoman?"

"Everything you're not," she snapped.

In second grade I told her about a project we were making in school. They were to be gifts for our fathers. Everyone was making the same thing, I told her, but I was creating a pin cushion in the shape of a chair, a more personalized gift for Dad.

"Yes, you would do that, wouldn't you?" she snarled. She really did, she snarled. "Why do you always have to be different? Why don't you do what everybody else does?"

I got the message: I just wouldn't do.

Whenever she was angry with me – which was often - she said she was going to "kill me." This made me very nervous. She said it like she really meant it, snarl and all. In her suicidal episodes, I had an uneasy feeling she might kill us both.

When I was a teenager she wrote a column for a neighborhood newspaper. She was an excellent writer. One time she showed me an article she had written. It was about me; how hilarious it was that I was fat. Horrified, I begged her not to publish it. She insisted she would. I ran to Dad. Thank goodness he came up from the basement and told her in no uncertain terms that particular article would be torn up and thrown in the waste can.

She was very invasive like that. She felt entitled to know every private thing about my life and if she couldn't ferret out from me she'd go elsewhere. She was especially peculiar about sex. She actually called one of my good friends and demanded to know if I was a virgin. Another time she told me I didn't have to make out with my boyfriends in a car; I was welcome to come in and do whatever on the couch.

Her confidences about her own sex life, which I did not welcome, made me very uncomfortable. She would tell me stuff like how much she and Dad enjoyed making love in the morning. It downright spooked me out.

On the other hand there were times Mom went out of her way to help me know how much I was loved. She'd write a name on a piece of paper and challenge me to write as many words from it that I could. She did endless crossword puzzles and shared with me her love of words. She listened to me when I was upset. She did volunteer secretarial work for Habonim so I could go to camp. She had her own style of doing things and at times she was delightful to observe.

Mom worked as an executive secretary for the Jewish National Fund. She disliked just about everybody there, especially the volunteers and her boss. The office was in our dining room so we were all privy to most of the goings-on. Mom would talk sweetly on the phone to some JNF muckety-muck, then the minute she hung up she'd spit out, "You Goddamned son of a bitch!"

Mom was also responsible for my love of dance. In fact, she was a former dancer. That's how she and Dad had initially met. He came to a B'nai Brith meeting and Mom was the entertainment. Her troupe performed a modern dance. Afterwards she was introduced to Dad.

When I read "Othello" one line of dialogue stuck in my head. It was Othello's explanation of why he loved Desdemona. "She loved me for the dangers I had passed," he said. "And I loved her that she did pity them."

That was Mom and Dad. Dad was forever grateful to her. He said she had taken a fouled-up, rough, mean son of a bitch and taught him how to love. Mom said he'd rescued and accepted her and gave her a life she could live. It made for a strong bond.

So dance was not only a love of Mom's, it had sentimental value besides. Sometimes, when we watched TV she saw me imitate various dancers. This delighted her. She would instruct me to dance in different ways – "do a flamenco dance, a tarantella, a waltz" – and I'd do it. It thrilled her to realize I had inherited some of her talent.

So off I was sent to Miss Ida's dance school where I learned to toe-heel-toe-heel and pirouette. But my love was always reserved for dancing free-form, just letting my legs do what I saw a dancer do, or to fill my body with the music and move in whatever way the music inspired me to move. It was odd. For all she discouraged me, Mom gave me confidence that I could dance.

In adolescence, after my self-esteem dropped five miles beneath the South Pole, I stopped dancing. I convinced myself I couldn't dance at all. I'd go to school dances and just stand there like a scarecrow. I wasn't so much a wallflower as a wall.

THE MYSTERY THAT BINDS ME STILL

One night I went to a party where the music was strictly Motown, tops in my book. I had assumed my usual statue position. My greatest fear, always, was that people would laugh at me if I tried to dance.

But when "My Girl" – my favorite song of all - came on, the beat and the upbeat lyrics were too good to resist. Cautiously, I moved onto the dance floor and wiggled around a little bit. I was so self-conscious I could barely take a step. Then my nightmare came true. A tall young man was pointing at me and laughing out loud. "Look at this girl!" he announced. "She's so scared about what she looks like, she can't dance!"

It was a moment of revelation and redemption as well. He hadn't said I couldn't dance. He had said I was so concerned with my appearance I was keeping myself from dancing. He was, I decided, correct. I cast off the cautious stiffness of wasted years, and began to dance. I became so well known for it that people who didn't even know me called me "The Dancer." I was filmed once dancing during a rock concert at Eden Park. From then on, dancing became my metaphor for freedom. It was my own sacred expression of joy. When the darkness inside me set in, dancing literally kept my feet on the ground.

In my early teens I had a break with Dad. He had supported – and taught me – the ways in which I rebelled, but as far as he was concerned I'd gone too far. Young gentlemen were pulling up in the driveway with their motorcycles to take me riding. This unnerved him. He would have liked it even less if he knew at what speeds we would go.

When Dad read a radical newsletter called "The Realist" that my friend Sue had given me, he declared it was obscene and I would never see Sue and Jerry again. As far as my parents knew, I didn't. I simply told them I was going downtown to the library and went to see Sue and Jerry instead.

I was a political activist in a number of causes, including the movement against the war in Vietnam. In the early part of the war Dad supported it and he was furious that I didn't. My rebellion startled him in other ways as well. I was getting a way too colorful mouth. I was bringing home all manner of tatter-clothed brightly-colored long haired friends. Dad desired them to cut their hair. Some of them, like me, were deeply into poetry. My poetic male friends were "a little light in the loafers," Dad said.

Our biggest break came over a relatively tiny thing – so I believed. My friend Ben claimed he had counted all of our friend Bruce's pubic hairs and confided in me the number he had found. I tacked this information onto my wall. Dad came in my bedroom in a spying expedition, saw the sign, and tore it down. Later he admitted he had destroyed my private property and he was wrong. That redeemed him a bit in my eyes. I memorialized Bruce's genital area again by putting up a replacement sign.

In the meantime, Habonim was getting crossed off my list. I had given it a lot of time and energy, including going to its camp. It wasn't like any other camp I'd come across. It barely had cabins, the cabins didn't have doors, and the grounds looked like a victim of World War Two. Before breakfast we worked in the gardens and did kitchen and bathroom chores. The idea was the place was run like a kibbutz. Nothing fancy – and in the philosophy of socialism. Everyone gave up unnecessary items like candy or extra money and put it in the *kippah.* Everyone took what they wanted and gave what they could; supposedly. Other than a lot of making out going on I don't know any rule that was violated as much as *kippah.*

I didn't fare much better at camp than I had elsewhere. Generally the people who liked me there were older and appreciative of my odd notions and creative mind. But amongst people my own age my social skills were zilch. I couldn't do small talk, didn't care for material things, was mad for books, barely knew what to do with myself and admittedly, behaved oddly at times. I wasn't particularly interested in make-up or clothing and that didn't endear me to the girls. None of these things were high on the acceptable scale of my campmates. I was aware of their disgust and they were aware that I was aware of it.

Except for the counselors, I couldn't tell if the purpose of the camp was to live an ideal or to find someone who would sit on your blanket with you for Friday night. Of course, I sat on my blanket alone.

On a mid-weekday it was announced a talent show would be held Friday night. One of the counselors, Adina, knew I could sing my lungs out and also knew I was looking for the lyrics of a very beloved song. It was "They Call the Wind Mariah," a real tear-your-heart-out-I'm-lonely kind of tune. That day she came to me with the lyrics and insisted I sang it in the talent show.

I couldn't imagine standing in front of all those people who held me in contempt and exposing myself to their ridicule. But my Mack Singer feistiness was calling so I did it anyway. I felt as ludicrous as I thought I would, seeing myself through those people's eyes. Then I opened my mouth and sang. I knew I had them in the palm of my hand. There wasn't a whisper in the house. When I was done there was a long pause, as if nobody believed what they'd heard. Then it came - the sound of absolutely thunderous applause.

I won the talent show and I had learned some lessons. I could earn people's respect, even their admiration, through my talent. It didn't change that they didn't like me but it made things easier, sometimes even more tolerable. It had also been my first experience with what I think of as the "Watch this" stance. It's a sort of dare-me attitude I exhibit as a defense when my feelings are hurt. In its feistier sense, it also invites anyone who doesn't like what I'm doing to shove it where the moon doesn't shine.

Every Friday night at home in Habonim we'd have Oneg Shabbat. It was a celebration of the Sabbath. We'd sing and eat and dance. I loved it. I was being groomed to go to Israel and I might have gone. But one Friday I brought a friend, a Methodist, to an Oneg Shabbat. I was told never to do that again. Non-Jews were not welcome. I couldn't believe their attitude. I asked them, weren't they being bigoted in the same way they complained about people feeling bigoted about them? It was a useless argument. Jews were Jews and then there was the rest of the world, according to them.

That was the end of Habonim. I couldn't condone such thinking so I left. The incident left me embittered and for several years I joined my father in the odd stance of being an anti-Semetic Jew.

In my early teens everything was happening at once. I had teenage hormones – which make every adolescent crazy – boiling around. My bi-polar disorder was surfacing. A.D.D. was assisting in the problems I was having in school. The stress of being elected my mother's caretaker and listening to her death-talk was taking its toll. The night before my fifteenth birthday it all imploded, formed a deep black hole, and I fell in.

I remember being excited about turning fifteen. I was going to have a party the next day. Suddenly, while I lay in bed preparing to go to sleep, my entire body began to shake. It shook for hours. I had no idea what was the matter with me. The shaking didn't stop until I became nauseous and threw up. Thus was formed the pattern, on and off, of the next four years of my life.

During each episode, every night I'd shake. Each time it stopped when I could finally throw up. Each morning I woke up dreading the day because it only meant night would come. And with it came the same unrelenting pattern.

During the day I was like an ice cube, or a wooden block. In this terrible box it seemed no one could get through to me and I couldn't reach out to anyone else. My one feeling was fear. I couldn't do or enjoy any of the things I did before. I couldn't read, watch TV, or listen to records. I'd just sit, still as a stone. I couldn't write anymore poetry. I became terrified to leave home. I found that I literally didn't feel like myself; I couldn't connect with the stranger that seemed to reside inside.

Thirty years later I would learn the two words that described where I'd been. One was "depressive episode" (it used to be called a "nervous breakdown.") The other was "depersonalization." It refers to exactly that disconnected, unreal feeling I had for all those years. I wasn't crazy. It was a genuine dysfunction of a depressive brain.

I also noticed that on sunny days I'd feel better. I'd ride the school bus praying for the sun to come out. Years later, too, I learned how sensitive bi-polar folks are to light, and how good the sun is for depression.

My biggest concern during this time was how to hold it together. I didn't dare let anyone know what I was going through. To truly be crazy

THE MYSTERY THAT BINDS ME STILL

– that to me was death. I'd do anything to keep people from knowing what was going on.

Mom and Dad knew, and later on, a very few friends. To hide it effectively enough I developed "The Mickie Act." This made use of my thespian talents so that I'd appear on the outside quite opposite from how I truly was. I found out much later that this masking is common for people with mental illness. You might see this in newspaper articles quoting the neighbor or co-worker of someone who committed suicide." But they were so cheerful!" or "they were so quiet," they'll say. "I'd never have guessed."

Well, if we knew then what we know now somebody would have noticed. Like my English teacher, who heard me remark how brave I thought people are who killed themselves; or the few friends who knew how neurotic I was. But for the most part I had The Mickie Act down pat. When later I revealed I was mentally ill, I heard those very words from many people. "I'd never have guessed."

In order to seem okay at school I carried on like everything was fine. I had a reputation for laughing a lot, and loudly. I was always enthusiastically invited to be in the audience of any funny play. Senior year classmates asked "What are you going to be?" I'd tell them a teacher or an environmentalist, when inside I felt my real options were to be in a mental hospital or to be dead.

Today I see commercials on TV about medications to treat all kinds of disorders. The disorders are described, symptoms given and assurances for possible healing or cures. Little happy or sad faces chase across the screen. I can only imagine what a relief it would have been to me then – to know I wasn't alone, that there were names for what I felt, that there were treatments to lessen its effect.

But that was then, this is now. As far as I knew I was nuts.

THE MYSTERY THAT BINDS ME STILL

CHAPTER FIVE: HOW TO FLUNK OUT OF HIGH SCHOOL

It's very easy. What you do is this: don't study, don't do homework, don't read any of the textbooks. When your mother looks in your bedroom or when you're in class, hold up the textbook with another book you're reading hidden within. Don't pay attention to what the teachers are saying. You don't have to have a low IQ; you can even be *very* intelligent. But if you follow these guidelines, by golly, eventually you will flunk out.

It may take a couple of years – it took me three and a half. Still, I kept up my grades in English. It was my favorite subject. I may have gotten F's in all my other subjects, but in English I had straight D's.

In the middle of my sophomore year I flunked out of Walnut Hills High. In January, I entered Woodward High School. By spring of that year, they had kicked me out. No one thought I'd ever graduate high school, least of all me.

Walnut Hills is the official Cincy Public's "smart kids" school. To get in you have to pass a test and have a certain IQ. In sixth grade when we took the thing we referred to it as "the Walnut Hills test." When I took it I was a nervous wreck. After all, there was that hideous "wreath" incident in kindergarten; who knew what horrors would be ahead?

I wanted to go to Walnut Hills badly, primarily because both Jon and Barry had gone there. It was an ego booster, too, to pass the test.

My brothers had long since informed me I was too stupid to pass it, so when I found out I had the angels played their trumpets and the gods danced in the streets.

Of course I signed up to go there, and went. I knew I was in for a challenge if for no other reason then WHHS kids had to take three years of Latin. Lord only knows what for. To be fair, it did help me out with vocabulary. But I really could have done without Gaul and its miserable three parts.

Latin led me away from all possibility of passing. By eighth grade it was obvious that I was never going to be able to read and write it. In seventh grade I loved the vocabulary and took to it like a scholar. But then the teacher had to start teaching us grammar. Grammar was my ultimate downfall, whether it be in English, Latin, or later in my pitiful attempt to learn Spanish.

I am convinced that I'm fine in conversational language. But grammar bores my ass off.

Walnut Hills was scary. In every class teachers lectured us about how we'd better do excellent work. Nothing less was expected of a kid at WHHS. We were not so smart; however, that we didn't have "ranges" of intelligence. There were the dumber classes – dumb that is, for a Walnut Hills student. I had some dumb classes and some smart classes and it was all terribly confusing. I was dizzy with being bright or stupid all day long.

THE MYSTERY THAT BINDS ME STILL

I was delighted by a student's comment I heard later on. "They tell you you're smart here," she said. "But you still be dumb."

Mary Jane Junk was my home economics teacher. For no reason I can think of she didn't like me very much. During the sewing semester she made me stay after school and work on my hopeless apron. She'd stand behind me and whine "With a name like Singer you'd think she'd sew like a dream." She even sent the apron to my guidance counselor as proof of my worthless work. During the cooking semester she let me stay in the kitchen long enough to eat dreadful stuff like minted grapefruit, but during cookie baking she threw me out. I had to sit foodless and uninspired out in the classroom for the rest of the semester.

In all classes the pressure was on. WHHS students *performed*. Matters were made worse by the legacy of my brother Barry who was brilliant, made all A's and had been accepted into one of the best colleges around. Much was made over Barry at home. My mother worshiped him. We all joined in Barry ideation. At one point I became so mixed up that I actually prayed to Barry rather then God.

My operating philosophy was this: I'm stupid. But I'm in a school where I'm not supposed to be stupid. So if I don't do any of the work, neither I nor anyone else will know I'm not able to do it. If I don't do anything and fail that's fine – because it's not really failure if you never did prove you couldn't do it at all.

Something like that.

This was neither an honest nor healthy way of thinking but it was all I could operate from at the time. No one knew about A.D.D. If teachers spoke in a monotone my mind went on with other adventures. I had no tolerance for boredom. It quickly led to depression. I was lousy at following directions. Rational subjects like Math would hit my head and bounce off. Tests were not my forte. I couldn't stay still. As far as most teachers were concerned, I was either stupid – or a bad kid.

The irony was, all the time I was flunking out I was getting one hell of an education. I loved to read. I was curious. I was a natural learner. I even *wanted* to learn about the doggone Hittites but I couldn't listen to the History teacher's drone. Every Saturday I'd go downtown to Pages and Prints, my favorite bookstore. I'd have two dollars to spend. Paperbacks were twenty-five or fifty cents then. I could pluck anything I wanted from the shelves. I loved history, non-fiction, fantasy, science fiction, biographies, plays and novels. I read everything from "Confessions of An Opium Eater" to Sherlock Holmes. These were the books that were hidden beneath my textbooks. I was making weekly trips to the library as well.

When teachers asked questions in class, it was often me with my hand in the air, ready with the answers – not the kids who passed all the tests. What I wanted to know I learned and retained. I realized early on that ultimately we were responsible for our own education. Neither teachers nor the subject matter they presented us with could make us learn. But a teacher who could spark her students, a teacher who could help them understand what learning was really about – could make all the difference in the world.

One teacher who demonstrated this was Mrs. Lorraine Kapell. She was my eighth grade English teacher. She obviously liked kids and her subject and she got genuinely excited when they learned. She delighted in getting them to think and watching them as they'd grow. She was anything but boring; I paid attention when she talked. She was more than a teacher for me, she was a savior.

I was *not* achieving academically, so it was inevitable an MDT (Multiple Disciplinary Team) meeting would be held on me. All of my teachers gathered with my mother and hashed over what a horror I was. My mother told me later when the meeting was over Mrs. Kapell, the only one who didn't bash me, asked her "Do you know what a treasure you have?" Then she said to me, "I've asked your mother and it's okay. I'd like you to come home with me."

And I did! I went home to a *teacher's* house! And sat at her dinner table with her husband and children and talked – like I was SOMEBODY. I was listened to with interest and respect. I believe there is no greater gift that can be given to a child than to be an adult who is not the child's parent – but who thinks that child is the neatest thing since sliced bread. Mrs. Kapell gave me that gift.

As another result of the MDT meeting it was decided that I would go to the school psychologist. And what a happy adventure it was.

I remember being given Rorschach tests, a series of smudged ink pictures. The psychologist held them up, one by one. Then she asked me what I thought they were. I think I was supposed to see something different in each one, but all I could discern was a multitude of bats. Then she gave me a "prompt" – that is, a drawing, and I was told to write a story about it. This was my forte, and I was prepared to shine.

The drawing was a depiction of a Victorian era-looking room with lots of plants and a housemaid was watering a very large one. I had been watching a lot of Alfred Hitchcock of late and was influenced by his tales. I took great pride in weaving an original story with a plot worthy of being used by Hitchcock. It was about a maid who hated her employer. The maid chopped her up and stuffed her down into the pot, cleverly concealing the crime by watering the plant.

The psychologist called Mom and told her I was psychotic. My poor mother was terribly upset.

Psychotic happens to be one thing I am not. This was also a lesson: I was to beware of the adults in schools who rarely listened to or understood the kids. This went for me when I was a student, and remained the same when I taught as well.

WHHS set me loose and I was sent to Woodward High School instead. This was a tremendous relief. There, kids were allowed to be as dumb or as smart as they chose. There were no more lectures on-go-to-college-or-else. The work was vastly easier – not that I did much of it, but at least I was churning out C's.

One Monday morning I walked in and the lobby was filled with black students, all sitting down on the floor. I asked what it was about. I was told this was a sit-in. The students were protesting what they thought to be an unfair expulsion of black students at another school. That sounded like something I could sink my teeth into so I sat down.

I was one of only two white students present. I was pretty visible. If that weren't enough, I got to my feet and opened my mouth a lot. Police and school administrators stood unhappily on each side of the lobby. I knew they had surely called Mom and Dad.

At three o'clock the school day ended and so did the sit-in. I walked home full of dread. What were my parents going to do to me when I got home?

Sure enough, they were waiting for me. I could see them through the glass in the front door. Dad wasn't in the basement, Mom wasn't at the stove. They were just sitting there on the couch staring at the door. I walked in.

Dad got up and moved in my direction. He lifted up his arms and I thought, get ready, here comes the blow. But he threw his arms around me in a hug instead then kissed me on the forehead. "That is for standing up for what you believe in," he said. "And by the way, I think you were totally wrong."

It was an amazing gift. He could tell me he thought I was wrong, yet still be proud of me for the reasons I had done what I did. In that moment he set me free. For good or for ill he recognized I had a mind of my own and I would follow it. He had taught me well.

One of the things Dad taught me was civil disobedience. For a man with his past, he had a strong appreciation for the law. He said that if a person felt by conscience he/she must follow a higher law, rather than legal law, then he/she must do so. But then, Dad told me, the law breaker must accept the consequences that came along.

It sounded fair to me. At the time I didn't know it was pure Gandhi and Henry David Thoreau.

My consequence was a ten day suspension during which the administration would consider whether I was to be expelled. They decided that since I was "troubled" I should have a second chance.

I hung in there and so did they but it wouldn't be the last time I was a handful. I walked out of teachers' classes if they made me mad. I challenged a school counselor about her authority. I complained to the administrators about anything I considered unfair. Automatic dial wasn't in existence at that time but if it had been Mom and Dad's phone number would have been at the top.

At the beginning of senior year the counselors sent each student's class standing to homeroom. Woodward High School was huge. 552 students made up the senior class. I opened up my notification. My class standing was 152 – which meant I was in the *upper third* of the class.

I couldn't believe it.

I went to the counselor's office and asked if this was her idea of a joke. "I didn't believe it either," she told me cheerfully. "But there it is."

Mom and Dad nearly fell through the floor. "How do you suppose this happened?" I said.

Dad considered this quandary and answered back. "It's clear," he said, "You're the cream of the crap."

Suddenly possibilities were opened to me. I could go to college. But what would I go to college for?

I've heard various clergy speak of getting a calling, a sure sign from the Lord that they're on the right path. I've heard it described as an inner voice, a burning in the soul. That's exactly how I felt the day I realized I wanted to be a teacher. Now my life made sense. If I loved learning I'd love teaching. I'd have the opportunity to do it the way I thought it should be done, not as most of my teachers had taught me. And besides, it was a great way to get a captive audience.

The desire to teach got me through a lot of difficult times ahead. I hung in there no matter what because I had a goal I wanted so much.

The first school where I taught was Walnut Hills.

The second one was Woodward.

Welcome back, Kotter. Welcome back, welcome back, welcome back.

CHAPTER SIX – ACCEPTANCE

By the time I was in my teens all I wanted was not to be the way I was. I thought of myself as monstrous in some way, or demonic. Whatever took me over felt like something out of "The Exorcist" – something dangerous and inexplicable; something that possessed.

F.D.R. said "We have nothing to fear but fear itself." He was absolutely correct. All it took was one panic or anxiety attack to bring on even more anxiety and panic about having another one. It was an endless cycle. Fear of the attacks ruled my life.

They started with a cold, frozen feeling in my stomach, followed by coldness all over, then a fear that overtook everything, physically and mentally as well. I was engulfed by waves and waves of anxiety that never reached a crescendo. With it came engulfing terror. I felt as if I would explode, or crumble, or crack. Wherever I was heading, it was something beyond death – it was the black pit.

The black pit defined might be craziness forever, or loss of self. But more than that, it was slipping into a place where only fear could live, and where no one could reach me, and where I couldn't reach out. Nothing terrified me more than that black pit. I'd do anything to keep out of it – if I could.

The pit grew over the years, growing wider and blacker still. I don't know if I could have traversed this darkness alone. I had the luck to have some extraordinary friends who stayed with me during the worst of it. They were people who accepted me right where I was. I clung to that acceptance as a lifeline, yet could barely grasp it, since I could not accept myself.

There were other things happening to me besides anxiety attacks. For years neither I nor anyone who knew me sensed that my moods were often extremely off-balance. I certainly didn't notice; I was simply used to being the way I was.

There were mornings I'd wake up and be immensely relieved because I could tell "it" was there. The "it" was a vast elation, a feeling of absolute intoxication with which I would greet the day. It was an ecstasy, an exhilaration, an enchantment. I was filled with an unspeakable joy. I loved every moment of life, felt everything was wonderful, and saw miracles everywhere. I was endlessly excited and couldn't imagine why everyone else wasn't experiencing life the same way. When I felt like this, I was grateful for being out of depression and assumed I was back to being my self.

I was magical. I was amazing. I was anointed. I was pregnant with bliss.

I was a creature of drama anyway – when this immense cheerfulness burst forth, everyone, including myself, assumed this was "just me."

It was not.

It was mania. Or more precisely in bi-polar two, it was hypomania.

I loved being this pied piper of happiness. I'd go out of my way to flavor other people's experience with the euphoria of my own. I'd sing, I'd dance, I'd write wonderful poetry. I was fun and charming and the life of the party. My students thought I was the happiest person they'd ever known. We'd stand to pledge the flag and I would be gushing with astonishment at how wonderful everything was. I'd giggle in delight.

When I was diagnosed with bi-polar disorder, no one who knew me believed it. They were used to the way I was; terribly depressed, immensely exhilarate by turns – sometimes all in one day. They thought of me as a mercurial personality. Even the therapist I was seeing at the time questioned it.

With all the symptoms of whatever I had, I never saw hallucinations or heard voices. I never thought I was Jesus Christ or the Queen of Sheba or anyone other than myself. In most people's minds, including my own, manic-depression (bi-polar) was a disorder solely for people who had experiences like that.

At this point in time, at least four different forms of bi-polar disorder have been identified. Bi-polar two is actually the version the majority of bi-polar folks have. It involves mood swings that go beyond the normal responses to something either happy or sad. The depression is darkness declining into the deep, the highs a rocket that explodes. Rarely is there psychosis, but judgment can be impaired; behavior can sometimes be a bit bizarre. Appetites of all types are huge – whether for sex or shopping or food or fill-in-the-blank.

THE MYSTERY THAT BINDS ME STILL

In bi-polar two of the highs are called hypomania because they are less extreme than the manias of bi-polar one. With bi-polar two bankruptcies are common. So is addiction. We will self-medicate what feels so unbalanced; sex, alcohol and drugs are the substances we use the most. Easy distractibility, intense rages and grandiose ideas of self are part of the package, too.

I have been through and exhibited it all.

I had food disorders that came and went as well. I either ate enormously and gained weight or became nearly dangerously thin. At one time I was borderline anorexic – before there was a name for what that was. I escaped drug addiction through my fear of lack of control. I escaped full blown alcoholism because I started to take valium and didn't want to mix them in a deadly result. I don't remember why I stopped taking valium. Happily, today I am neither drinking nor taking addictive drugs.

Not knowing that I was bi-polar, I also didn't know bi-polar disorder could involve ungodly rage. I found that from the day I began swallowing effective medication my rages totally ceased. Until then they were horrible. Just ask my son.

David, who I had when I was in my thirties, became the focus for all my rage. I have not resolved my guilt about that. When the anger took over I know I was literally seized by something that was not myself – but I still must live with the fact that it was out of my body and out of my mouth when that monster raged.

I didn't hit David, so I thought I wasn't abusing him. But I was. When I was in a rage I don't know where "I" went. What took over was a madwoman – irrational, screaming, throwing things, kicking doors, beating on the walls, threatening, exhuming an anger so fearful and consuming it scared the shit out of me. It was utterly uncontrolled; once it came I couldn't stop it. I had to go with it until it wore out.

I can only imagine what it did to David.

I could never bear to watch the television show called "The Hulk." I *was* The Hulk – the raging giant green monster that rose out of an otherwise ordinary person, so big, so frightening, with the power to kill.

Oh yeah, that was me.

I've described this phenomenon to some people who have told me they just don't believe it. Cute little four foot ten me – Nah. They couldn't even come close to picture it in their heads.

Bi-polar rage is a horrifying thing. Readers of Stevenson's "Dr. Jekyll and Mr. Hyde" or viewers of any of the movie versions would know that. That novel is a perfect portrait of bi-polar rage. Make no mistake; I may seem to be no more intimidating than a flea – but when the rage took over I could make Mr. Hyde look good.

Everything about me would change. My ability to think. My control. Even my voice. It was like being consumed by a fire so hot all I could do was fuel the flames.

THE MYSTERY THAT BINDS ME STILL

There were times when I was absolutely, totally nuts. I cannot believe some of the things I did. Here's one of them:

This occurred when I was a "professional", a "grown-up" an intelligent (usually kindly) person with common sense. I would no more think of being rude or making unreasonable demands than I would think of eating my head. But I was in the midst of a bi-polar "episode."

It was winter and I was deep into my depressive mode. I wouldn't get dressed, stayed in the house, wouldn't talk to anyone but my husband. I felt as frozen as the weather outside. It was Christmas holiday so I wasn't teaching, which made it worse. Even in my worst depressions I often got a lift from the kids.

My comfort, my self-medication, my addiction was, and still is, food. I looked to that for some cheer. On that day I learned that Wendy's was advertising a new sandwich. Ah, I thought. The very thing.

It took a great deal of energy to motivate myself. I would have to actually get dressed, get in the car, and get out of the house. I made it to Wendy's, gave my order and came home, eager to have my fix. I opened the wrapping and discovered what I had was not what I'd ordered. To my vast disappointment it was just a common cheeseburger.

My disappointment quickly turned into rage. I called Wendy's and demanded to speak to the manager. Then, in the words of my husband, I proceeded to tear her as a new asshole. I screamed and yelled and carried on. When she suggested I return and I would be given a free sandwich that only made it worse. It had been so hard for me to get there in the first place. I went into a frenzy, raving at her "What do you expect me to do *now*? Just what do you expect me to DO?"

I got nowhere because of course there was nowhere I could go. But five minutes after I hung up I was still raging. I called that poor woman and did the same thing *all over again.*

I was a different person when I was "bi-polar gone." I'd do odd things that didn't make sense. I'd burst into sudden tears at a party. I cried endlessly or couldn't cry at all.

It was worse when I couldn't cry. I would wake up sad or mad for no reason, and have the feeling of water trapped behind my eyes. At night, instead of being able to sleep, my mind would run like an engine out of control, thoughts spinning in a loop that wouldn't end. All of this may not have meant I was crazy, but it was crazy-making. Inside there was this person, me, where I didn't want to be at all.

I didn't know that I was being ruled by imbalances of chemicals in my brain. Half the time I was so used to the constant up and down, I didn't even recognize there was anything peculiar going on. There were times when people remarked about how fast I talked or noted that my moods would change all the day (I'm known as a rapid cycler) but nothing seemed different about it to me. I just figured I was emotional, highly dramatic and often just out of my mind.

In talking with other people who have bi-polar disorder, I've found they share many of the same experiences. The most painful thing, we all agree, is the aftermath of an episode. How do you apologize? How do you make it right? How do you explain that "that just wasn't me"?

It's more complicated than it may seem. From my experience, you can say you're sorry and do what you can to make amends, but more often than not the person whom you have wronged still views you as nuts. And "nuts" can mean everything from out-and-out crazy to inferior to simply unacceptable, or all of the above. Sometimes you may not have wronged anyone, but simply have exhibited some sort of questionable behavior. Try explaining your "strangeness" to someone who doesn't believe you or understand.

I had that problem in several situations, but especially in the high school where I taught for ten years. I had good friends there but many members of the faculty concluded I was – take your pick - odd, rude, and/or inappropriate. There were a variety of reasons for this, including that I was apparently monopolizing the teachers' phone. I really wasn't aware of it, but I was. I was on the phone because I was trying to keep it together. If I felt like I was going to crash, the best way I could take care of that was to make contact with someone who knew me and understood what was going on. Without such validation I could get worse. I didn't want to, nor could I afford to, walk into the classroom in the grip of an episode. In order to seem "fine" when I had to function, no doubt I was on the phone a lot.

At one point I decided I'd do what I could to correct the negative impression I made. I went to several faculty members and listened to them tell me why I wasn't liked, and then I'd try to apologize and explain. It was humiliating to find myself telling them I was really a *nice* person, really I was.

Once I got my diagnosis there was relief in learning that I *wasn't* crazy – I was just mentally ill! I had a zillion flashbacks to past events. For the first time I could say "oh, so *that's* why it happened, or *that's* what it was." Just a little bit, just a smidgen, I could let myself off the hook.

But not very much. Guilt, self-condemnation, and shame had been my partners all my life. I survived in part because of the people who knew me and loved me, no matter what. They were my rescue, my blessing and my saving grace.

One of these people was Jody.

I met Jody Sussman in my gym class, tenth grade year. The first day we sat on the bleachers next to each other (both of our names began with "S"). We didn't know each other, but read what we wrote on our parental referral cards. We were supposed to give our full and correct information.

I had no intention of giving any such thing. Where I was to provide my father's name, "PANCHO GONZALES," is what I penciled in.

THE MYSTERY THAT BINDS ME STILL

Jody was charmed and delighted. In that instant she became my best friend.

Jody shared in my appetite for nonsense and mischief and a little bit of larceny, too. She listened to me and loved me. We were together all the time.

She was one of the very few who knew what was really going on with me. It didn't make the slightest difference to her. Jody enjoyed my sense of whimsy and my humor, and if I was in pain she was there for that too.

Jody's first memory of me is when I asked if she wanted to take naked pictures with my friend Camille, me and her boyfriend Harold. "Harold shakes a little bit when he sees a naked woman, but he calms down." I assured her. "It'll be fun."

I have since asked her why she continued be friendly with me after this startling invitation. "Have you ever watched a train wreck?" she said. "It's deadly, but it's fascinating."

High school was just awful, boring, depressing, dragging on and mostly a waste of time. Jody and I brightened each other's days. She tolerated me beyond comprehension. Once when I was crying she gave me her sleeve for a handkerchief. I wiped my eyes and – not thinking - blew my nose in it as well. She screamed, but barely flinched.

In turn, I was very protective of her. On a St. Patrick's Day we came to school dressed as leprechauns. Admirably, it was Jody's idea, and she really put herself out making her costume. She rigged a pair of turned up elfin shoes, which were quite painful to wear. Jody was relieved to remove them after school. I walked with her while she was barefoot to her locker and down the hall.

We were followed closely by two rough looking big hulking guys, walking just behind. I heard one of them say, "Hey! That girl's barefoot! Let's stomp on her feet!"

Without a moment's hesitation I whirled around. "You stomp on her feet and I'll stomp on your balls!" I cried. I jumped up as high as I could and I punched the young man in the nose. I doubt that it hurt, but it certainly did take him back.

Jody and I were partners in mischief. She would do things like walk into a classroom and spontaneously hug some unsuspecting boy. Once she did this over a teacher's strenuous objection. "Jody!" he yelled. "Have you no manners?"

"Yes, I do" replied Jody. "I thanked him."

The only time Jody lost patience with me is when I went into my flower child mode. One night I told her, "There are stars in my nose. There are stars in my nose…. There are stars in my nose."

'Shut up or I will *punch* you in the nose," she told me. I knew she would do it, too. Jody was spunky as hell.

Jody's background wasn't rosy. Her mother was a single mom, tired, and overworked. Her once-husband didn't want children and stopped speaking to her when Jody was born. Jody never met her father and maintained she never wanted to. The family wasn't well off. They lived in a tiny apartment and rarely ate dinner. The dining room table was covered with hair-curlers and make-up instead. Jody's mother believed when life was tough you had to get tough to live it. She taught that to her daughter, too. When she took on two jobs Jody was ten. "I'm through being Mommy," she told Jody. "I can't raise you anymore. From now on you're on your own."

Our allegiance to nonsense was the best remedy to depression we had. It was like medicine for me. Playing had energy and joy; it affirmed life, especially when I couldn't affirm much of anything about it.

Jody was also there when I was in the grip of Obsessive Compulsive Disorder, the most paralyzing disorder I've ever had. Rituals haunted me, things like having to read every sign and piece of trash I saw, sometimes over and over again. It was in many ways more frightening than my panic attacks. I felt as if I was trapped in a cycle of appeasement to some cruel gods whom I never could please no matter what I did. Even more than depersonalization, it robbed me of my entire sense of self.

But Jody could still make me laugh. She hated to see me holed up all the time so she took me for walks. I trusted her implicitly or I wouldn't have gone. There were so many signs out there I could stand there reading them all night. But Jody was patient and gentle. She'd pause while I read a sign and wait. Quietly she'd ask if I was ready to move on. If I wasn't, she'd wait without complaint until I was.

No matter how bizarre my behavior was, Jody never thought I was crazy. She believed in me and accepted whatever came along. If I had to read signs, I had to read signs.

Her support kept me going, I have no doubt of that. I can't imagine having gone through that without her.

Camille accepted me totally as well. She was as gentle and loving as anyone I've ever met, with a sweet nature that reached down to her soul. We ran around barefoot in parks, daydreaming and giggling a lot. I felt so safe with her that at a time I was afraid to leave my house overnight I could manage to spend the night with her. It became a Saturday night ritual. I'd come over, her ill-tempered Southern grandmother would bitch; we'd eat fried chicken and okra and cook kettles of fudge.

One Saturday night Camille invited our friend Michele over as well. The three of us piled into her big bed. I was feeling scared that night, afraid I wouldn't get to sleep and that would result in an anxiety attack. Not only were the attacks miserable, but once one started, I was afraid it would never end. But Camille reassured me enough that I closed my eyes and fell asleep. In the morning when all three of us woke I discovered I had wet the bed.

"Eeeeeeeew!" said Michele. "You wet the bed! How could you! That's so disgusting!"

At the same time Camille spoke as well. "Mickie, that's wonderful," she said. "That means that you must have slept."

Someone cared for me so much she could handle that I *urinated* on her. I still marvel whenever I think about it. I don't know if I could have done the same for somebody else.

Jon's girlfriend Eileen brought her sister Carol over one day. I was fourteen and Carol was twenty. Despite the age gap we became good friends. At first it was dicey because Carol's father didn't approve. He was a wealthy businessman and an Orthodox Jew. He'd heard rumors that the Singers were pretty wild.

But when he came to pick her up one day he noticed my father was wearing a yarmulke, a Jewish skull cap, on his head. After that he told Carol she could come over anytime. He was impressed. "Any man who wears his yarmulke in the house is okay with me."

In fact, my father could have cared less about Jewish religious rules. At Passover when he'd lead us through the Haggadah (the prayer guide) he'd skip huge portions of it at a time. "This is mere conjecture," he'd say. Carol's father didn't know that his yarmulke served a purely secular reason – it kept our parakeet from scratching the bald spots on his head.

I was on the phone with Carol one night when I felt a peculiar sense of "leaving myself," something that happened to me from time to time. Hard to describe, the sensation felt like my mind was floating away. I had no idea this was an "episode." I assumed this was just another step leading to the black pit. I told Carol I didn't feel right. "I feel like I don't know where I am."

Someone else might have told me I was nuts and hung up. But Carol didn't treat me as if it was odd at all. Very gently she said "Then let's find you" and began with reminding me I was sitting on the bed in my room. I knew that, of course, but just then nothing felt real. Carol literally grounded me and like Jody and Camille, she didn't back away at times like these.

Such friends were my manna from Heaven. They gave me something to hang on to, a sense that there was something worthwhile about me after all. They were miracles – they were angels.

THE MYSTERY THAT BINDS ME STILL

CHAPTER SEVEN: AN UNLIKELY LOVE STORY

Love amongst lovers was something I knew nothing of. I looked at romance from the outside, barely a bridesmaid, never a bride. Whatever brief liaisons I managed lasted at most a few days or a week or two. Neither I nor the gentlemen I attracted had much staying power. I was, however, the champion of dating males with odd names: Ivars Villums was one, Whelocke Winspear was another. But my favorite was Jackson Two Trees.

One Saturday afternoon I gathered with friends for a "happening" in a concert hall. We sat on the floor in a circle, locking arms and chanting "om." We did it with gusto, giving it a wide voweled "ah-ohohohohohoho" and then bringing it on home with a definitive "mmmmmm." After a while we modified it by being the sound of the wind: "whoa-ohohohoh-ho-ah-whoooooo." After about an hour we took a break. I scrambled into a giant-sized rocking chair and settled in. Suddenly a boy leapt into my lap. He was skinny, limber and entirely serious. "I am Jackson Two Trees!" he announced. "And you are a lost Indian princess who I have looked for and loved for 2,000 years!"

This was news to me and I told him so. I had a heck of a time extricating him from my lap. He whooped and twirled around the room crying out his claim: "I am Jackson Two Trees! You shall be my lover again!"

Believe it or not, I gave this guy my phone number. I figured he said he loved me so who was I to argue? I was definitely hard up.

This burgeoning relationship lasted one phone call. Then Jackson Two Trees disappeared. Undoubtedly in another 2000 years, we will meet again.

I longed for a relationship, but gave out the message "stay away." Even my wardrobe was rather threatening: sweaters, mini-skirts, chain belts, a Cockney hat and stomp-on-me leather boots. I wanted – but was scared of having - a boyfriend. My heart may have been yearning but my clothing and body language said "approach at your own risk, and prepare to be doomed."

Still, I did have some openings and invitations. In high school I was approached with flirtatious greetings such as "What's happenin', little mama?" I even took lessons from my friend Tony as to what flirty sorts of things I was to say in return. There were three possibilities: "Nothin' to it," "S.O.S." ("same old story" or the tangier "same old shit") or my personal favorite, "It's all you, baby." But I didn't have the nerve to go through with them. Some boy might actually take an interest and what would I do then?

I'd had my crushes, however. My biggest one was on Jon Abts.

I met him in eighth grade at Walnut Hills. He was walking down the hall, a vision beyond belief. This was early in the sixties and very few people in conservative Cincinnati were wearing any unusual clothes. But Jon was straight out of a

THE MYSTERY THAT BINDS ME STILL

Partridge Family David Cassidy wet-dream. He had long brown hair down to his shoulders and love beads around his neck. His blue jeans were practically painted on; his feet were sheathed in brown leather boots. I took one look at him and thought: either he has to be the coolest boy in school and he doesn't care what anybody thinks – or he's the weirdest boy in school, and he doesn't care what anybody thinks.

It turned out that he was the weirdest boy, but I didn't care. I was nuts about him.

We got together, but with my usual luck, only as friends. I wanted more but I was used to the good buddy role and resolved to be a good friend. That year Jon was going through a hard time. He was a Methodist minister's son and he had reached his time of rebellion – no longer did he want to be the good little boy. He dedicated himself to getting into as much trouble as possible, and I enthusiastically supported him. At year's end, however, he ran away from home, left Cincinnati and didn't return. Such was the abrupt end of my crush on Jon Abts.

Three years later he called me. I was 17; he was 18, and he was back in town. He wanted to see me that afternoon and gave me an address in the worst part of the city. Then he gave me a warning: "You might as well know," he said. "I've changed a lot. I've spent the last three years as a biker."

Frankly I was a little scared to see him. I didn't know what I'd find.

Jon had, in fact, changed a great deal. I found him much rougher. Morality no longer seemed to concern him. His rebellion had gone beyond where any rebellion of mine had ever been. We had a cautious visit; the kind of uneasy time old friends spend together when there is little left to bind them as friends.

It was winter and darkness came quickly; it seemed a good idea to get out of that neighborhood. So I said goodbye to Jon and made my way down his beer-smelling stairs.

Up the other side of the stairs my worst nightmare was approaching.

It was a young man – he looked to be about my age and he was not very tall, but he didn't have to be. His shoulders filled the entire stairway. Every part of him bulged and rippled with muscle; every inch of him was covered in black leather. Weapons hung from every part of him where anything could hang, huge tire chains dangling from his pockets and his neck. Most startling of all, he had *no hair*, just a strip sticking straight up in the air like a Mohawk Indian.

Twenty years later I had students with this hairstyle. Punk rock had come and gone. But *nobody* looked like that then.

If I just ignore him and keep climbing down the stairs, I'll be fine, I thought. I wasn't counting on him whirling around and grabbing my wrist. He pulled me to his side. "Where do you think you're going?" he demanded.

"Home," I said in a quavering voice.

THE MYSTERY THAT BINDS ME STILL

He studied me a while, then broke into a slow smile. He nodded his head to the negative. "No, you're not," he said.

He turned me around and pushed me back up the stairs, right into Jon's apartment. (It turned out he was Jon's roommate.) Then he led me to the couch.

He pushed me down and stood above me, hands on his hips, legs drawn apart. "Hi, I'm Traveler," he announced.

"Hi, I'm traveling," I answered and tried to get up off the couch.

Traveler pushed me back down. This time, he said nothing. Silently, he moved his hands to his belt, slowly removing it, and sliding it to the floor. Then he thrust his thumbs in his pants, moving downward.

I closed my eyes. I screamed. Was this the rape my mother was always warning me about?

When I opened my eyes, he was still there. Fully clothed. On the floor was a pair of black leather pants. He pointed to them. "Those are just my snow pants. I was out *sledding*," he said.

We both laughed and he sat down next to me on the couch. For the next two hours we talked. After a while I began to notice other things besides his weapons and his Mohawk hairdo. I began to notice he had the sweetest, gentlest, tenderness blue eyes I'd ever seen.

It was the beginning of my first real relationship.

It lasted all through the school year and into the summer. Not that it was always on a smooth course. It's not that we fought; it's that Trav was never "tied down." He chased anything that wore a skirt. If we encountered each other when he had another female the rules were I was to say hello and butt out.

It was a raw deal, and unforgivably chauvinistic to boot, but what Trav gave me, and what I gave him, was something special that transcended traditions and rules. I wouldn't stand for such behavior today. The truth is, neither one of us could sustain a more committed relationship than we had.

It wasn't a conventional relationship; Traveler never even asked me out on a date. Mostly, we tended to "hang out" and know when and where we'd probably do the particular hanging.

When we first got together, everyone who knew us was perplexed. My friends couldn't imagine what I was doing with this biker; his biker buddies couldn't figure out what he was doing with a Jewish virgin. We were considered a *very* odd couple indeed.

But they didn't understand.

Traveler was born half German-American, half Indian, in a bigoted, small Texas town. Everywhere he went he was called "half-breed" and other nasty names. As he told it, he was twelve years old when he had had enough. He stole a Harley-Davidson motorcycle and left town; never to return. He missed the half of childhood he had robbed himself of.

THE MYSTERY THAT BINDS ME STILL

And I was the Hippie Queen. Everyone knew that. I told everybody that if I *bothered* to graduate from high school I was going to hitchhike out to San Francisco, where I'd make my living singing and playing the guitar on street corners. Of course, I didn't even know how to play the guitar. But Trav knew that.

Both of us had worked hard for survival. Both of us had long worn and wearied of our "tough guy" masks. When we were with each other we could be who we really were. For both of us, this was a new concept in a romantic relationship.

Nothing we did fit other peoples' expectations of what we would do. The biker and the Hippie Queen smoked no grass nor had wild sex. I posed on top of cars wearing his clothes; he played with my naked toes. We dipped our feet in streams, held hands, went swinging, giggled, kissed as often as possible and played in any way we could.

We used to hang out in Clifton, a "hip" Cincinnati neighborhood. We especially frequented a rot-gut neighborhood bar called "The Firefly Café," although we had no business being there since both of us were only seventeen years old.

In the sixties everyone lodged themselves into categorizes, drew tight circles around who they considered enemies and who they considered friends. People were either "hip" or "straight," a "dove" or a "hawk," over thirty or under thirty, a member of the counterculture or a member of the establishment. It was highly divisive; few people lived in the in between. If different groups were together they often clashed. Such was the case at the Delmar Bar, just across the street from The Firefly Cafe. The denizens were hawks and definitely members of the establishment. If I or my friends walked in we were hooted at and summarily told to get out.

But at The Firefly Café, everyone was welcome. It was a cultural oasis. It didn't matter if you were a hippie or a politico or a student or a Republican, a pot-smoker, a beer drinker or a bum – as long as you spread the love, you were welcome.

Gloria and Jean, the owners, liked liveliness around the place. They were often hostesses to The Animals, Trav's biker gang. They liked it when I came in because I'd dance. As soon as I came in the door, Gloria would yell over to Jean, "Put a quarter in the jukebox! She's here!" And they knew just which song to play: "Hot Fun in the summertime" by Sly and the Family Stone.

Smokey was a six foot 10 inch biker who weighed about 120 pounds. He hung out at the Firefly Café, and "Hot Fun" was his favorite song, too. More times than not he was there when I was and the two of us would end up doing "The Funky Chicken" all over the place.

I was hanging out with bikers, handing out condoms at the Free Clinic, and otherwise hob-knobbing with fellow misfits of society. It felt free, open and innocent, not like in the pot-smoking circles I had put in the past. The people I met were often surprise packages; stereotyping couldn't predict what they would do. One night that I sang at a coffeehouse was particularly memorable. Suddenly it was overrun with The Iron Horsemen, as serious a biker gang as they came. I was terrified to open my mouth, much less choose music they might want to hear. So I thought "here goes," and sang a rousing program of gospel songs. They loved it and so did I - here was a room full of self-proclaimed outlaws bouncing around and clapping to "Will the Circle Be Unbroken" and "Carry Me Home."

It was the season that would be known as "The Summer of Love." As far as I was concerned, it was.

It was such an amazing time that it didn't take much for Trav and I to have interesting experiences. For a while we worked at a 24-hour crisis phone service, where a group of Hare Krishnas had unnerved us by crashing through the door and hollering up the stairs. They surrounded Trav and I. They were chanting "Hare Krishna, Hare Hare" over and over which seemed to have no end. From then on we locked the door and when the bell rang, checked out who was standing there before we let them in.

So one day when there were two men ringing the bell, we didn't automatically open the door. We looked out the window and checked them out. They had short hair and were dressed in gray suits; this was not a common sight in the neighborhood. Per standard operating procedure, we asked who they were.

"Open up," they answered, "It's the FBI."

From that point on Trav and I got very excited. We were so thrilled we forgot to keep our cool. We demanded to see their badges and giggled when they took out their notebooks and pens. They took down our names and all I could think was "wait 'til my mother hears about *this.*" They asked if we knew the whereabouts of Mark Rudd or Bernadine Dorhn. They were revolutionaries far out of our league, known for bombing buildings at Columbia University. Trav and I just looked at each other and laughed. Know Mark Rudd or Bernadine Dorhn? Who, *us*?

We may have known how far we were from that world; it wasn't so clear to the FBI. I don't know about Trav, but I got an FBI file out of it, fifteen pages long. I still have it. Most of the pages are headed by my name and then covered with huge patches of opaque black ink. The black coverage, they wrote in explanation, was meant to protect national security. I don't know what they thought I was doing but it must have been powerfully dangerous stuff. On the last page they conclude I was just a kid with a loud mouth of no threat to anyone. I could have told them that. Their agents could have been busy chasing after the bad guys and saved their country a lot of black ink.

For Traveler and me, it was the best summer of our lives.

THE MYSTERY THAT BINDS ME STILL

At summer's end our fates began to take a turn. I *did* graduate high school; I was going to college. To be a teacher, I hoped. Traveler's main agenda was to get hold of a Hawg. We were in different worlds, and our differences split us apart.

Two semesters into my freshman year it was New Year's Eve. Just for old time's sake, I went to the Firefly Café. I walked in and there they all were; all the Animals. Jake, Smokey, Peanuts, Squirrel, Snake. And Trav – he was there too. He had dressed up for the occasion in black leather, so polished that it shone. And he had decorated himself especially, ringed with a large boa constrictor wrapped around his neck. He saw me and asked me to dance.

I asked if he would mind removing the snake.

We danced, ate, talked and danced. Suddenly back at the table Trav got quiet. He just stared at me, and then he got up and stood in the doorway, staring at me some more. It was an odd, electric moment that caught everyone's attention. Everybody just hushed, staring at Traveler, staring at me. And then he spoke.

"I love you, Mickie," he said – and then he walked out that door, and I never saw him again.

After that, I talked about Traveler to some folks almost as if he was a story I wrote, not someone I'd really known. I talked of him to my husband this way, too. In the years since Trav had walked out the door, I had gone on to become a high school teacher, then a graduate student, a college instructor and a wife. I had taken my husband's name and was listed by "Mrs. Scott" (well, sort of; a name change is being employed).

I was hired at a small branch of the University of Cincinnati in the countryside, far from the outskirts of town. It was primarily a school for adults working to earn degrees while they already had established jobs. When I realized I was going to be out of town the first week of scheduled class, I asked a colleague at UC if he would mind taking over for me for the one class I would miss. I asked him to have the students write letters to me telling me all about themselves.

A week later, ready for my first class that night, I read through the stack of letters that had been left for me. Of course, none of my students knew who I was, only that I was the yet-to-be-visible Mrs. Scott. The letters were fairly unremarkable for the most part, although one had a name that sounded faintly familiar scribbled at the top. I couldn't quite place it. It was written by a man who wrote that he was glad to be in higher education because he had never finished the education he had before. He wrote that he'd been in Cincinnati briefly before as a teenager and he was glad to be back, now with his wife and son. He went on to note he was glad to be in a more civilized life altogether, having had a wild youth that began when he stole a Harley-Davidson and took off from his home state of Texas…….

I thought, no. It can't be him.

I had a list of the home and work phone numbers of all my students. This man was employed at General Electric. I called GE and asked for him by the name he had written at the top of his paper, and got him on the phone.

"Hi," I said. "I'm….Mrs. Scott, your English instructor. I know we haven't met yet, but I've read your letter and I think…it's possible we might know each other. Would you mind if I asked you a couple of questions?"

"No," he said, "go right ahead."

"Okay." I breathed in. "Um - did you hang-out in the "hippie" neighborhood called Clifton?"

"Yes," he replied. My heart was beginning to flutter.

"Okay, then," I said, "Did you frequent a bar called The Firefly Café?"

"Oh, yeah," he said.

"Uh…" I took another breath. *Did you wear your hair in one strip going up the middle of your head like a Mohawk Indian?*"

"Yep, that was me," he laughed.

"Then Traveler," I answered. "You'd better sit down. 'Cause this is Mickie."

There was a long silent pause at the other end of the phone. Then he spoke – always a rather commanding sort of guy, he hadn't changed, because the first thing he said was, "BE AN HOUR EARLY TO CLASS."

I said goodbye to my husband, told him what awaited me, and drove out to the college. I sat there waiting for him, behind my teacher desk. Then – there he was, standing in the door. I would have recognized him anywhere. He wasn't in black leather anymore – he was wearing a gray suit, and a tie. And he had hair. But his shoulders still filled that doorway, and he still had the sweetest, gentlest, tenderness blue eyes I've ever seen.

He strode in through the door, grabbed my shoulders, and picked me up off the floor. We threw our arms around each other in an enormous hug.

And that began the worst summer of my life.

Because the course I had signed up to teach was "The Theme of Love in Literature," and every poem, every play, every novel I taught that summer all had the theme of love, passion and romance. And there I stood at the head of the classroom, the acknowledged expert on all of those things, and no one – except for one – knew that the one who had taught *me* those things was sitting right there, in that room.

THE MYSTERY THAT BINDS ME STILL

CHAPTER EIGHT: THE PSYCH WARD

High school was over for me in 1970. In the fall of that year, college began.

Like many teens, I was in no way prepared for life beyond high school graduation and all that it would mean. Even though I disliked it, high school was an anchor. Like most students, I had my friends, my reputation and my well defined "place." No one among the thousands of University of Cincinnati students cared that I was the Hippie Queen. I was just another face in a humongous crowd.

To make matters worse, all the classes I took had hundreds of students in them and took place in Wilson Auditorium. I arrived at the auditorium at eight a.m. and stayed until three, generally falling asleep in between. Meantime Math, Psychology, Philosophy and Geology had all floated by, entirely unnoticed by me.

Eventually I began to realize my behavior was getting pretty weird – even for me. I was in a downward spiral, closing further and further in on myself and isolated from the rest of the world. I felt more and more "unreal."

I became afraid to talk to anyone. This was highly unusual, given that I fed on people and talk. When I was in the cafeteria, I held my head down so I wouldn't see anybody I knew and feel obligated to say hello. I holed up in the library most of the time, reading poetry in the small poetry room. Or I'd slip into a study carrel, where if

I leaned far in, the two privacy boards would hide me from everyone else.

It got weirder yet.

I started bringing large umbrellas with me when I went to the auditorium. These I would set up in front of me so that no one could see my face.

After a year of this, I suspected something was more wrong than it had ever been before. In short, I thought I was losing it.

So I set about trying to save my life.

Whenever fear got the best of me, I used my "pull yourself up by the bootstraps" approach. A few years before this a friend of mine had invited me to stay with her and her family on an island in Maine. But I couldn't do it because I couldn't leave home overnight. Of course I wanted to go but I knew I couldn't and I didn't want anyone to know why. I told her I would come, though, thinking that at the last minute I'd pull out.

It went so far that I actually packed my suitcase and waited for her parents to pick me up. I knew that when they knocked on the door I'd just apologize and tell them I couldn't go.

But when the knock came my iron will did, too. "Alright," I said to myself. "You're right. You *can't* go. But your feet can. Get out of this bed and move them."

And that's exactly what I did. I felt quite disinterred, as if my legs were separate from the rest of my body, and certainly from my mind. My feet kept moving, and they moved me out the door. I spent three unforgettable weeks in Maine.

THE MYSTERY THAT BINDS ME STILL

I could do something like that again, I thought. I could force myself sane.

I was faced with two major difficulties: I couldn't talk to people and I couldn't stay away from home. My solution to this was to take a job as a camp counselor the following summer, where I'd have to talk to people, and where I'd be two hours away from home. I would make myself do what I couldn't do and then I'd be back to myself again.

That was the grand plan. At first, although it was unnerving, it was fun. All staff had to report to camp a week ahead of opening so that we'd be taught things the kids would be taught to do. This included horseback riding and boating and city girl that I was, doing these things was an unprecedented thrill. I learned how to row a boat. I loved it. I took one out on the lake one day after the kids had arrived, quite a number of who were in the water at the time.

Not long after I took off I got my left and my right mixed up, and despite frantic calls and whistles demanding that I turn around I couldn't figure it out. I headed straight for the roped off swimming section, and the kids. The lifeguard had to get them all out of the water, and I was forbidden to take out a rowboat again.

I was made song leader and had a ball getting everyone to sing. I was also seeing my first snakes, and my first ticks. One night I played a recording of Mary Martin singing in "Peter Pan." I couldn't hear it very well so I turned the volume up to the top. It was ten o'clock at night; all the campers had been put to bed at nine and were presumably asleep in their beds. I hadn't realized the record was playing over the P.A. "I'm flying! I'm flying!" was blasting all over the camp. In some ways, I was having a good time.

But at night the shakes came and the dread, which often carried over to the daytime. I was talking to people but it was still a strain. I didn't feel safe; I wanted to go home.

But I wasn't going to let myself go home. I employed my old trick. Our beds were iron cots with a bar in the back. I'd lay there and tremble and think "I can't stay here. I can't." Then I'd answer myself right back. "That's true," I'd say to my weaker self. "You *can't* stay here. But your hands can."

I'd throw my arms behind me and grip the iron bar until my hands turned white. The shakes came and went and the sweat broke out on my forehead. I believed I was going to overcome my craziness with this surefire method: just make yourself do physically what your mind can't.

I did this for six weeks. Intermittently I made sand candles and hiked through the woods and danced whenever Carol King's music was played over the P.A. I was doing what I always did – keep functioning, keep moving, keep a smile on my face.

Until one day I couldn't do it anymore. I began crying and had no idea why. For three days I cried, some off, but mostly on. My junior counselor had to take over for me. Day and night,

THE MYSTERY THAT BINDS ME STILL

I stayed in the cabin and cried. Finally I called Jody, who said the obvious: "Come home."

So I did, telling the camp director I was having a "nervous breakdown" – or so they called it then. When I got home I was like a zombie or a ghost. I was there, but not.

What happened next had to do with my least favorite family story of all. When I was a little girl the family had a dog, a beautiful black Cocker Spaniel. Everyone loved him, including me, but I did a little girl thing to him. Dad had me loving black olives, just as he did. This dog had an inviting black nose with two holes in it; it looked to me like a shiny olive. In curiosity, I stuck my fingers up the poor dog's nose. Naturally he took exception to what I had done. He bit me.

That did it, apparently. Mom and Dad got rid of the dog. And I took the rap.

Jon was the most upset. He called me "dog killer" and never forgave me – not for a long, long time. Animals mean a lot to my brother. They touch him in a place he otherwise reserves for children, and whatever he cherishes in his life. Getting rid of the dog truly broke his heart.

Mom gave me "The Message" again. The dog wouldn't eat unless she was with him, she told me. Wherever he was he would starve now and die.

Not only was I a bad girl, I was a killer. I could kill my dad and now I had killed a dog.

When I returned from camp in my zombie state, Mom decided she would cheer me up. *She surprised me with a black Cocker Spaniel puppy, just like the one we'd had.*

In my extremely vulnerable state, it was the worst possible thing anyone could have done. It's not that I don't like dogs; I do. In fact I love them, puppies most of all. But I couldn't handle having to take care of one. It stirred up all my bad girl feelings, all my guilt about being a killer. To be given a dog that looked exactly like the dog I "killed" sent me over the edge.

The puppy was cute; I held it and petted it, threw up and shook.

Whatever had allowed me to function up until then was no longer there. I was gone.

Elvis may have left the building – I had simply *left*.

Thirty years later I found out what was wrong. I had gone into a severe "depressive episode." I had my own term for it. I had fallen into the black pit.

Mom took me to the psychiatrist I was nominally seeing at the time. He said I should go to the psychiatric ward and signed me in.

It took a long time for the beds to be cleared and the papers to be signed and whatever else. Meantime I sat in the emergency room thinking "This is it. I've gone crazy. This is the end."

Jon was an intern at that same hospital. The intern who took me up in the elevator was Jon's friend. I knew him and liked him. And now I was crazy and he was taking me to the place crazy people go. Of all people, why did he have to be my escort? I was relieved when he left me with a nurse.

The nurse unlocked the psych ward doors, which opened and locked with finality behind us. I turned to her and said: "I don't think we're in Kansas anymore." She looked at me as if I was crazy, of course.

But I didn't care. In that moment, I had a flicker of hope. If I still had a sense of humor I was still in there. I wasn't totally lost.

I was in a different world in the ward, both literally and figuratively. The doctors asked me to name the president of the United States, and recite my phone number. It was downright alarming. They were acting as if I had no mind at all.

It made me mad, too. The doctor concluded his examination (which I later realized was to establish if I were lucid) and asked me what I thought they could do for me in there.

"Not a damn thing," I said, "if you're going to ask me questions like these."

There was a clear boundary between patients and staff there. It was palpable – I could feel it. What it amounted to was "You're crazy – I'm not. Keep out." In other floors of the hospital, staff tended to you, doing whatever they could to help. They certainly didn't look down on you because you were ill. They had open and friendly attitudes. Such was not the case among the staff attitude in the psych ward. They were aloof and patronizing, as if they were afraid that what we had was catching and they didn't want it.

The first thing I noticed is that the ward was run like a prison. There were rules and regulations up the gazooie and there were punishments, too. You could be confined to your room for any infractions, which I managed to do. The psych ward provided the term that at last described me. The word was "inappropriate." I heard it there a lot. "Miss Singer, you are being inappropriate," they'd say. It was a handy definition – it kind of put being a bad girl, crazy and a killer all in one efficient word.

The best thing about the psych ward was the other patients. Unlike the staff, they were not judgmental. Some of them were even fun. Most importantly, we spoke each others' language. There was no hiding and no shame among the patients. We provided hope for each other, and if not hope, the feeling that at least we were all in this together. For the first time I didn't feel alone. It was the patients who provided whatever healing that occurred.

I made the mistake of laughing when a nurse handed me a "Genuine Bard Clean Catch Mid-Stream Urine Collector." I thought the name was hilarious. I still do. The nurse told me I was being inappropriate again.

I made The Bigger Mistake the day we went to Proctor & Gamble. Don't ask me *why* it was necessary to transport 30 mentally ill patients to P&G, much less how the staff conceived it to be a good idea. But when you're in the psych ward, you do what the big guys tell you to do.

THE MYSTERY THAT BINDS ME STILL

Here's the way it went: at 6:30 a.m. a nurse entered my room and said, "Wake up, Miss Singer, and get dressed. You're going to Proctor and Gamble."

Then she left the room, leaving me totally perplexed. Did P&G have a psych ward we were being transferred to? Were we to be enslaved to make soap? Why would a nurse wake me up abruptly with this information with no explanation at all? Something very fishy seemed to be afloat.

I got dressed and sat down at the dining area to eat breakfast. Next to me sat the ward supervisor, the Big Nurse. I turned to her and said, "I find it rather amusing to be awakened when I'm in a psych ward and told that we're going to Proctor & Gamble."

The nurse looked penetratingly at me with her large blue eyes. "Well, Miss Singer," she replied, "*I* don't find it amusing, but I'll be glad to sit here and listen to why *you* think so."

If ever there was a time or place when one truly questions one's sanity, it's in a psych ward. Her response to me was frightening; I needed a reality check. I went down the hall and grabbed some patients, telling them the story. "It *is* funny, isn't it?" I asked.

They reassured me that it was.

So we all piled into cabs and went to P&G. We were taken to an auditorium where we were shone a film on how P&G made soap. Then we left. We didn't even get any samples of soap – the staff was afraid we'd eat them.

I suppose it was considered therapeutic to get us out in the world. Our next field trip was to a football game at the University of Cincinnati. The Bearcats were playing somebody and a group of us (along with staff of course) sat down in the bleachers. I knew absolutely nothing about football. In fact, I know nothing about any sports, don't watch them and don't go to see them – except nowadays where the exception is tractor pulls and demolition derbies at a place called The Buck.

There was a good looking guy in the ward, my age, and schizophrenic. I was quite taken with him. He went in and out of reality but it made no difference to me. He'd talk about his very own comet and his happy trees and I didn't care if he was psychotic or simply imaginative. I found him utterly charming. He liked me as well so we sat together at the game.

The game was not a good experience for me. I knew they took me to it so I'd have some entertainment, but I had no idea what those guys were doing down in that field and my mind started wandering into depression. To deflect this, I thought I could ask my friend to explain to me about football. He was male. All males known about football.

But he had slipped off his reality-base. When I asked him "What's going on down there?" He replied, "The grass that isn't GREEN! The grass that has NO MIND!"

That's all I know about football to this day.

THE MYSTERY THAT BINDS ME STILL

My affection for my friend caused My Biggest Mistake Of All. I visited him one day while he was in the bathroom brushing his tongue. While I waited for him, I laid down on his bed. Fully-clothed, and non-seductively: there weren't any chairs in his room so I waited for him on his made bed. A nurse walked by and was apparently stunned. Her eyes widened as she cried out" Miss Singer! Come with me *at once*!"

I was confined to my room. Nineteen years old, a college sophomore, but I was confined to my room.

It was heartbreaking, listening to the patients' stories of what had brought them to the ward. There were several nurses who were patients. One of them was in for drugs; I remember another one had poured Drano down her throat. There were assorted suicides and one very angry woman who went in and out of psychosis quite a bit. They'd lock her in an enclosed room where she'd shout "Jesus, they're cutting off my leg! Jesus, they're cutting off my leg!"

Two patients who remained friends after we all got out were my roommate and "the reverend." The instability of his marriage had put him into depression. My roommate had post traumatic stress disorder (another one they didn't have a name for then.) The night of her wedding her fiancé was killed in an automobile accident. She was having horrific nightmares and flashbacks. She dated everything with the date of that night. Her pain was excruciating. Every night she'd scream like somebody was killing her. She'd roll around so wildly in her bed that I often had to call the nurse to get her head out of the bars.

We all had two sessions with a psychiatrist, art therapy and a couple sessions of group therapy. None of it was the least bit comforting or helpful. But I look back with affection to my fellow patients, every one of them fighting their private hells to get well.

All of this happened over thirty years ago. I hope that today they do a better job. The hospital did then, and does now, have an excellent reputation. But there's been a long and widely held stigma against the mentally ill, sometimes even among health professionals. In insurance, in care, in affordable medication and therapy, the people with mental illness are often at the bottom of the pile. It doesn't surprise me that this hospital excelled in everything else and did such a poor job treating those with mental disorders.

Many people are afraid of mental illness, and of the mentally ill. They don't grasp that it's widespread, that anyone at any age is susceptible to it, that it's not emotional weakness but a real biological medical condition. They don't realize that a diagnosis of mental illness is not necessarily a description of someone babbling on street corners. And if there *is* someone babbling on street corners, the person watching generally is repulsed. They do not see there is a person in there, simply in the grasp of an illness.

Our language is full of derisive slang toward mental illness: "out-to-lunch, elevator doesn't go all the way up, doesn't have all their oars in the water, loony-tunes, and crackers, nutty as a fruitcake" and so on. Today, if someone on television was to utter derisive language toward an ethnic group it wouldn't be allowed. In our educational facilities, stereotyping is discouraged; bullying is too. Yet you can turn on any show on TV – cop shows especially – and you'll hear all kinds of derogatory terms for mental illness – "psycho" appears to be the favorite.

Check out the merchandise of a t-shirt vendor and look at the slogans on the shirts. More likely than not, you'll see a lot of these: "I only do what the voices in my head tell me to do," "I brake for hallucinations," "I'm proud to be psychotic," "Don't take away my delusions – I enjoy them" etc.

They're not funny; they go beyond rude or not politically correct. They're cruel. I know a lot of people who, if they had done what the voices told them to do, would be dead.

Much of the same kind of thing shows up on bumper stickers and key rings too. For all of these, I have some slogans I'd like to suggest:

"Cancer is to die for," "Leave me alone, I'm in a diabetic coma," "Tuberculosis takes your breath away," "Kids, be organ donors: play in the streets," "Get HIV – share a needle with me," just for starters.

Of course such slogans would never appear anywhere; it wouldn't be tolerated. They're not funny. They're cruel; they are reminders of the horrors in life. Yet making comedy out of mental illness is considered perfectly alright.

There's a big difference between being mentally ill and having a sense of humor about it and being someone who simply treats this often life-threatening condition as something to laugh at. Ask anyone who has gone through it, or anyone who has a loved one or family member that is afflicted. One in every four Americans deals with mental illness at some point in their lives; equally, those many families go through a hell of their own. Like alcoholism, it can become a family disease, causing unhealthy dynamics and depression that can develop as a result of watching a loved one go through their disease.

The stigma feeds the stereotypes, and the secrets. I kept my condition from friends, family, co-workers and employers. I didn't want anyone to know. Too many times I had heard the mentally ill laughed at or treated as inferior. I felt threatened that I could lose a job if my employer knew. And I sensed the fear people had about mental illness; the distance they tried to set between "them" and "us."

I have used what some consider derogatory words in this book, such as "crazy" or "losing it" or "nuts." I have done so because in those years those were not only the terms, they expressed the prevalent attitudes. I was terrified that I had turned into someone "crazy," which meant someone to look down upon, who would be reviled, and could never succeed.

However, if you're personally dealing with mental illness, you'd best be prepared to laugh. You'll need it. Laughter is healing. If you're living

THE MYSTERY THAT BINDS ME STILL

with a mental illness, you're living a life that is, at times, absurd. No one has the right to insult you or put you down. But it's valuable for you to know what your own sense of humor can do for you. When absurdity is tempered with a sense of humor, it can be a saving grace.

The psych ward did not provide what I needed therapeutically, but it did give me a rest away from the world. I was there for ten days and never heard a word about what was wrong with me, or even if there was anything wrong with me at all. I was given the phone number of a psychiatrist I was to see twice a week, put in a cab, and sent home.

Mickie R. Singer

CHAPTER NINE: COLLEGE AND OTHER HORRORS

I was fresh out of the psych ward in my sophomore year. As far as finding my place in college life, I was still utterly lost. It helped that I was taking some literature courses in the more intimate spaces of classrooms, but I had a hard time paying attention. This was probably due in part to being rather out of it, and in part because most of my instructors bored me to death.

Unlike teachers, college instructors are not taught to teach. They're chosen for their academic standing and their publications. Some of them happen to be wonderful teachers anyway. Some are not; they have no teaching techniques other than standing behind a podium reading from notes. Some of them only want to teach graduate students, or prefer being scholars, and don't like students at all.

If I was in an instructor's class who spoke in a monotone, I went to sleep. I carried around huge 30 ounce cups of coffee to sip from, but they didn't help. The coffee made me nervous and I still went to sleep.

But then I met Michael Atkinson and life in college was never the same.

Michael was an English professor and the best teacher I have ever had. He was humorous and dramatic, knew his literature, helped us to think, and was unbelievably smart. And he had a sweet little ass.

THE MYSTERY THAT BINDS ME STILL

I deeply appreciated it whenever Michael turned his back to write on the board. Those quick viewings lifted my spirits considerably. I soon found out that there was another student in the class who appreciated Michael as I did, all around.

She and I became good friends and between her and Michael I began to feel more at home. One day Michael and I inadvertently created a real life drama. Mom, who was willing to support some goofiness now and then, had made me a monk's robe, or at least a facsimile of one. I had a thing for monks' robes; I thought they were mysterious, and I had a very brief romance with a gentleman who actually was an ex-monk.

I wore it to school. On one occasion when I wore it I was late to Michael's class. Softly, I tapped on the door. "Ah," I heard Michael say, "It must be Friar Tuck." He opened the door – and there I was.

Michael became a friend. He introduced me to Marx Brothers movies, for which I am eternally grateful. At one point he was in charge of bringing in the poets for the English Department. Michael would invite me along to dinner or wherever he entertained them. For someone who loves literature, it doesn't get any better than that.

In one of my "lit" classes I had a particular problem. The professor had chosen such horribly depressing material that halfway through the course I came to him and confessed I couldn't read another one of his books.

I had gotten involved with the Women's Center and had my own key, which made me feel like hot shit. We made banners and tried to get the female students roused up, but UC was a very conservative school. They didn't rouse easily. So we left them alone and roused ourselves and had fun. I did a lot of Mae West imitations, and for a while the Women's Center was home.

I hung around, too, with what was left of the revolutionaries. I was offered the presidency of the SDS (Students For A Democratic Society, who had turned into rather a radical group.) Wisely I turned it down. Two of us took a course called "Politics of Protest," which was taught by an instructor who disapproved of protest in any form. It was also inevitable that eventually my friend and I would begin to protest. We did, and got thrown out of class. Even though we both had A's, the professor gave us "C's" – because of our conduct! This was unheard of, especially in a college. We appealed it but got turned down.

Such ventures were a wisp of what was left of my former days at "The Independent Eye." The Eye was an "alternative" newspaper in Cincinnati – our news was concerned with reporting supposed police abuse and what new band was coming to town. Stuff like that. I wrote prodigiously, loved the paper and loved the people who worked on it. We tried to be very serious, but didn't always pull it off. Traveler worked on the Eye for a while, too. It was my most "radical" time. To paraphrase Shakespeare, I was full by a lot of sound and fury, which added up to mostly nothing.

THE MYSTERY THAT BINDS ME STILL

Working at The Eye brought me to my first actual brush with the law. I was innocent, however, which they eventually figured out.

At the end of that summer, The Eye and I had parted ways. The staff had sunk to a few people and I had disagreements with some of the few who were left. At that time The Eye was located in a tenement. I had painted it and fixed it up, and decorated it with some of my posters. When I left I still had my stuff there, figuring I'd retrieve it some other day.

Shortly thereafter The Eye office was firebombed. My posters and such burnt in the fire. When I got the news I was sorry to hear it; my stuff didn't matter all that much but I was sorry for The Eye.

My sorrow was nothing compared to what happened next.

The police called my house and accused me of doing it.

When my father got on the phone and vouched that I'd been home the night before they dropped it. Years later, there was an investigation into suspicious acts by police during the sixties. It turned out THEY had firebombed The Eye! Supposedly they interviewed some neighbors who fingered me. When all this came to light I was able to read the actual police report. Sure enough, I'm described as the perpetrator. Get this:

They reported that I had arrived at the Eye house, driving a sedan. I jumped out and climbed onto the roof with accelerants. I set the fire and jumped down. Then I drove away.

This was pretty interesting stuff, given that I didn't know how to drive (I didn't have a car or learn to drive one until I was 23 years old) and obviously lacked the considerably athletic ability to climb or jump off of roofs.

Such was my brush with crime. As my FBI file concluded, I was not a wrong-doer. I was spirited and I had a big mouth. That was about it.

During college I had my first actual date and it was a doozie. I had a crush on this guy I kept seeing around. He worked at the Free Clinic and had long blonde hair and a beard. What the hell, I'll call him Poindexter. If he knew it would annoy him immensely.

I wanted to meet him and one day I saw my opportunity. I was still working at the phone crisis service, which was directly across from the Free Clinic. Next to the clinic was a small park where I spied Poindexter walking his dog. Immediately, I asked my boss if I could borrow his dog and off I went to the park.

In the sixties, we encouraged each other to be playful and uninhibited. The idea was we were the gentle generation. We practiced free love and free speech and protested because we cared. We were not embarrassed to be seen skipping down the sidewalk or blowing bubbles in our backyards. We danced with abandon. We were supposed to be full of life.

As in any decade, there are behaviors that are considered "cool" and behaviors that aren't. Back then, that was the expected behavior, and even if you didn't feel like it you acted like you were full of joy.

I wanted to impress Poindexter so I was prepared to be one hundred percent full of joy. I put the dog on a leash and commenced bouncing and skipping joyfully around. I got his attention, alright.

"Hey, lady," he said. "You'd better watch out. You've wrapped your dog around that tree!"

My first attempt didn't go so well. But I kept at it, and after a few months, Poindexter asked me out on a date. A real, grade A, genuine American date!

I wore clothes that night designed to make me a knock-out. Poindexter was impressed. "Wow," he said.

We had dinner and then went to the opening of a new nightclub. I was just three days short of my 18th birthday. The bouncer looked at my student card and said, "Nope. Sorry, Poindexter. She's too young. She can't come in."

Gentleman that he was, Poindexter went in without me and got good and drunk.

I was left standing alone on the sidewalk. But I didn't feel at all abandoned and I was not upset. The whole time I waited I just kept thinking, "Wow. I'm on a date. I'm really on a date!"

I look to that incident today to reassure myself my self esteem has come a long, long way.

Despite this disaster, which I was too clueless to mind, Poindexter and I continued to see each other. Poindexter thought it was just terrible that I was a virgin, and thought he was the man to do something about it. He believed himself to be quite a ladies man. He said that as far as women were concerned, "I fuck 'em first and get to know 'em later."

I was so naïve I thought that was charming. He badgered me continually about my virginity. He wasn't the first to do so. Being a virgin in the sixties was simply unimaginable amongst those who preached free love. I wasn't having any sex, yet my friends were tumbling in and out of lots of beds. I was even appointed the watch-out at times. I got to the point where I was just heartily sick of the whole thing.

So one night I phoned Poindexter and said, "Alright already. I'm appointing you – I want to get rid of my virginity."

Poindexter was absolutely overwhelmed. "No one has ever called me – just called me out of the blue - and said this to me! I can't believe it! You've got to be kidding. This is outrageous."

"Well, believe it," I replied. "Now are you going to do this or not?"

"Okay," he said. "When do you want to do it?"

"I have to get birth control pills...I have to take them for at least a month...." I made a date for five weeks ahead.

On the appointed night I reported to Poindexter's apartment. It was accomplished. With cold detachment on his part, and no pleasure on my part. But I was satisfied. I had gotten rid of the doggone virginity. Now, for once, I could fit in. I could say to people: "No, I'm not a virgin." Those were the golden words that made you hip, grown-up, and groovy to boot.

After that, Poindexter and I had no interest in seeing each other. This didn't particularly disturb me. I had gotten over my crush and he had annoyed me enough with his badgering that I was ready to move on.

It was years before I realized why Poindexter didn't want to see me anymore. He prided himself on being a man who used women whenever and however he could. I didn't realize it then – but I had used *him*! It must have been a heck of a blow to his ego. I call it poetic justice.

I had about a year and a half of getting my bearings at UC and then I got sick again. I had developed Obsessive Compulsive Disorder - OCD. Per usual, I had no name for it nor did my psychiatrist give me any understanding. I really don't know if psychiatry was at that time so uninformed, or if I should have been told things that I was not. All I knew was that suddenly I was a slave to rituals and obsessive, overwhelming thoughts.

Reading signs and trash as many times as my brain commanded me was frustrating and terrifying. There were days when I could do nothing but my rituals. I couldn't get past my front yard. There were also days when I couldn't leave the house at all. I remember one time some friends came to visit and we all sat on the front porch. I had to go read the trash on the ground – I had to do it. But I didn't want to miss their visit, or have them see what I had to do. I gripped my chair tightly and stayed put. I could barely breathe and my head felt like it was on fire.

Many of my rituals were public, and those were the most difficult – and shaming – for me. I feel uncomfortable about them even now. One took place in my neighborhood right next to my house. I had to straddle in the window of Kotter's Hardware Store and look at all the merchandise, slowly, left to right, until whatever ruled me said I could stop. This took place in front of neighbors and anyone who was passing by.

At school, I was driven to do a ritual in a history class. I had to walk to the other end of the classroom and touch the thermostat. Then I sat down in my seat. About fifteen minutes later I had to do the same thing. The professor and the students were not kind about this. I was the butt of nasty comments and jokes; I was also shunned.

I didn't want to leave school; I wanted to become a teacher. My psychiatrist was able to work out a deal with the college for me to be considered a "special student." This meant that I could stay in school, but I could only take one or two classes per semester. For this reason it took me five years to complete college rather than four.

To help people understand how OCD works is pretty impossible. It has a "how" but it doesn't have a "why." I can't explain the "had to" of my rituals. It doesn't make sense, but there it was. Something in my brain misfired and I was stuck in an irrational loop. What made it worse was having these rituals for no apparent reason. I never understood why I was particularly compelled to do some things but not others, such as to repeatedly turn off faucets but not have to keep washing my hands. It felt TRULY crazy. Not being able to stop it made it seem even crazier.

I had to look certain ways at the moon at night, touch faucets over and over again, had to leave food on my plate, and so forth. Once when I refused to read a sign I was thoroughly punished. My body trembled, my head felt on fire and I couldn't breathe to such a degree that I had to take a bus all the way back to where I'd seen the sign, read it and then take a bus home again.

OCD is scary stuff. I felt afraid all the time because the message my brain was giving me was that I was unsafe. Always unsafe, unless I followed the rituals. Yet performing the rituals only made me feel safe for a while. Once done, a ritual would still have to be repeated; immediately or later or over and over again – it was different every time I was driven to do one. As a result, I was *never* safe. What waited for me was worst than death; what, I couldn't say. Perhaps even worst than the black pit.

During this period I had the part of an Irish landlady in a college play. I loved doing it, hamming it up, finding a costume, developing what my father called "bits of business." I was particularly proud of my walk, which the director also admired. He asked me how I'd developed it. "Easy," I told him. "I pretend I have a dump in my pants."

But to do something I enjoyed, I paid the price. My inner demons punished me and my rituals became more pronounced. The irony was, I appeared so nerveless and in control that my fellow cast members called me "The Iron Butterfly."

They had no idea that every night after rehearsal I'd fling open my front door and run like hell down the hall to the bathroom. I didn't want to vomit on the carpet.

At times people around me thought the rituals and compulsions of my OCD were an amusing quirk. They were not – they were hell. It is difficult for anyone who has not had it to understand. OCD robs you of your freedom to be your own person or to own your own life. It can happen to anyone; financial or social status makes no difference. Successful and famous people can – and do – have it as easily as anyone else. It is a cruel and terrible place to be. Observe an animal in a cage; see it pace back and forth, back and forth – look at its haunted eyes, its desperate demeanor, its aspect of fear and despair. You are looking at OCD, and it's nothing for anyone to enjoy.

I went through several years of this, then gradually it subsided and the severity of it disappeared, thank God. It was the worst of any illness I ever went through. I still have a mild version of it. I honestly don't know how I'd handle it if it fully came back again.

When I came out of the OCD, I had Michael to help pull me back to life again. I took every class he gave. Sometimes they were so intimate we would all meet sitting on the floor in his office.

THE MYSTERY THAT BINDS ME STILL

In one class on Eastern Religion, not only did we all become close friends, 5 different couples came out of it and several marriages. And one of those couples was me and my first real boyfriend.

Another one of the couples was Michael and my friend from several years ago. They married, and I spent a spring and summer with my beloved. It was a very good experience for me; he was a sweet guy – and playful, like Traveler. But it was short-term. The break-up hit me very hard; I mourned him for the rest of the year.

Student teaching kept my head above water. I thought I would love teaching but I was enjoying it beyond anything I'd ever imagined. I was working under my savior of the past, Lorraine Kapell, and I was teaching at Walnut Hills. Lorraine gave me free rein from the start, so I was the only teacher the students were used to. No matter what was in the curriculum I found a creative way to teach it, something way "out of the box." It was a love fest. The kids did well, they loved me, and I loved them. While I was working with them we established a new literary magazine and made a record (a 45). I also got the kids to paint Lorraine's room and I painted a design on her window, which got me in trouble with the principal who had told me not to. But my arrogance was boundless back then, and it would be quite a while before "I learned."

I also helped establish the Thursday Lunch Bunch. One day I brought in candles, a tablecloth and flowers and arranged them on the table where Lorraine and our group would be sitting. Everyone liked it. It was a touch of elegance, something to make a difference in our day. So we pledged to do it every Thursday. After a while we had themed lunches. One was for the art teacher who we insisted was going to be bar mitzvah-ed. We toasted him with grape juice and then I pulled out a paper cutter. It was great fun to see his face.

The kids and the teachers got together before I had to leave, and they proclaimed a "Mickie Singer Day." It was announced over the P.A; the students gave me a booklet they had all written in, and I got cards and presents all day. Given all that I'd been through to get there, it meant more to me than they could ever have known.

I was able to pay my way through college because back then it was fairly cheap and I worked whenever I could. The jobs I had became an important part of my education too. To pay for my freshman year I was a nude model for an art school. I figured I had the guts to do it and it was preferable to my last job, making pizza. Plus, I was used to it because my mother was an artist and I was often employed as a model for her – clothes on.

When I arrived at the school I was given a brown robe and guided to the dressing room. I took off everything but the robe, climbed onto the platform, dropped the robe and assumed a position. In the next few seconds I was staring right into the eyes of a guy I had graduated with the year before. What else could I say but "Fancy meeting you here?"

THE MYSTERY THAT BINDS ME STILL

I modeled for painting and sculpture. Somewhere in the universe there's a canvas or two floating around with my image on it. The art teacher was an old curmudgeon who told the class "What's the matter with you? Draw her as she is. I get you a model that looks like two ton Tessie and you paint her like she's starving to death."

Two-ton-Tessie wasn't particularly pleased with that remark, but I needed the job. I stayed there up until the day some student ruffians decided it would be fun to throw clay at me. I let them know my mama didn't raise me to be their human target, and left.

My next job Jody got me. Jody had been raised a Catholic but was now working at an Orthodox Jewish School. This upset her relatives. So they told her about a job opening at the Convent of Mary Reparatix baking communion wafers or altar bread – I forget how they are referred to first. Naturally, Jody called me and said "Have I got the job for you."

I was given an interview immediately with Sister Ida. I told her straight out that I was Jewish and she said she didn't care. I was hired.

I am forever grateful that I had this job because it's so much fun to tell people about it. But the work itself, frankly, was boring. We'd all have certain jobs which would cycle each week. One job was making the dough. Now *that* was a genuine thrill. You had to pour lots of flour in a five foot vat chased by gobs of water from a garden hose. Then you spread a heavy plastic cover over the top, flicked on the switch, and held on for dear life. It lasted for nine bone-shaking minutes. When you were finished, you had a new appreciation of being able to stand on your feet.

The next job was distributing the batter in bowls. Someone would dip big ladles in the dough and fill up large silver bowls. These would be taken to the bakers.

The wafer-baker machines resembled waffle irons and the principle of making them was the same. You threw a ladle of batter onto the iron, which had round or fish shapes. The oven is closed for one minute; things steam, you open it back up and voila! – you have produced a thin sheet of fried dough with communion wafer shapes in it.

The last job was pressing the shapes out and sorting through them. If any of them weren't perfect – if a piece had been broken off – we were allowed to eat them. Unblessed as yet they were just fried dough. The flour and water batter served its holy purpose, but the wafers they did not taste particularly good. Yet sometimes we'd get so bored we'd eat them anyway.

The garbage cans where we worked had wheels on the bottom. I climbed on top of one of them and rode around the kitchen. The other ladies did not like it. They called Sister Ida who forbade me to do it again. I stayed on the alert, though, for any entertainment that wasn't forbidden. One day I looked out the window and saw a young man. He was dressed in blue jeans and was naked from the waist up. His hair was long and curly and he was quite tanned. I asked the ladies of the kitchen who he was. "Don't *tell* me he's a priest," I said.

"That's Larry the gardener," replied one of the ladies in a disapproving tone.

It was time for my mid-morning break so I ambled over to the yard to introduce myself. "Hi, I hear you're Larry the Gardener," I said. "I am Mickie the Wafer Baker." We didn't form any romantic ties but Larry would often take me home in his truck, which was nice of him. The only drawback is he spent a lot of time making anti-Semetic remarks. I doubt he knew I was Jewish. He'd turn to me and say, "Gotta go over to the Hebrew Union College and cut the grass. Damn Jews. You know what they're like."

I was amused to find out that whenever I took my mid morning or afternoon breaks, the ladies thought I was out having a quickie in the garden with Larry. Truly, they over estimated me.

I also went over to Hebrew Union College (HUC) but not for the purpose of cutting the grass. It was a school for rabbinical students, who at that time were still mostly men. They had given Jon free room and board there in exchange for his budding medical skills. For a little while at that time, about a year, Jon and I were friends. I'd come over and visit. I was big on baking and bringing him cookies. But I had another motive as well. The rabbis - to- be didn't see much of the opposite sex and they were the horniest group of men I have ever known. Any time I wanted a lift for my feminine ego, all I had to do was go over there and allow them to try and pick me up. I wasn't ripe for any picking, but I appreciated the attention.

I suppose, on some sort of moral scale, it's fitting that I was a nude model and a communion wafer baker next. I can't say that I've entirely behaved myself in any of the jobs I have held. I doubt I ever will.

THE MYSTERY THAT BINDS ME STILL

CHAPTER TEN: MY LIFE AS A SEX BOMB

Okay, so this will be a short chapter.

I'm probably no more confused about this body-image thing than most women are. I think a lot of men are confused about it too. It astounds me how much dithering we do about our body parts: this part is too small, this part is too big, this part is too round, this part's not compact, this is too short, this is too tall, this part sticks out too much. This part doesn't stick out at all.

When you break it down, that's what it's all about.

I've grown up with an assortment of "body image" beliefs; everything from "don't judge a book by its cover" to the pop culture message that if you don't look like a model or movie star you might as well give it up.

My Big Truth, handed down from my father, was that it was a woman's job to be a visual treat for men. I took it very seriously.

As an adult, I have been up and down the scale with enough numerals to fill the universe. Pick any number between 95 pounds and 185 pounds and I've been there – probably at least twice. I refer to my various body fluctuations as "incarnations," that is to say, different selves.

At age 22 and 95 pounds I was way too thin, but I didn't believe it when people said so. I looked gaunt and pale. I was terrified of food and kept a tight rein on whatever I ate. Half of a hard boiled egg for breakfast felt like too much. Lunch was vegetables; dinner was vegetables too. If I ate anything more than that I'd feel so guilty I'd throw up.

I lost the interferon needed for a healthy immune system. For years I got every cold and virus that came along. I'd get low fevers that sapped my energy and lasted for months at a time. But I thought it was all worth it. I had become a visual treat.

I wore skin tight jeans and painted on tops and flashed a little low-cut style too. I was doing what I believed I had to – to get a man, to please men, to fulfill my father's and America's ideal.

I traded being called a "wide load" to being referred to as a "hot mama." Both of them felt uncomfortable; neither of them fit my idea of me. I knew that a few months' eating habits could make the difference between either designation. It was confusing when people responded differently to my changing shapes. It was still just me, the same woman the pet store owner flirted with when I was slim, and the one who ignored me the next time I walked in – fat.

My boyfriend in college lived in a house with three other guys. I loved it. We'd cook, we'd eat, and we'd wrestle. I was one of the boys. For a long time, that was the most comfortable I'd ever been. Being a woman was scary stuff. When I dreamed, I was a male. I was finally convinced I was a woman when I had a child. I knew only the female gender could do that.

I have a photograph of me in a bikini on the beach. I was cute and curvy and weighed less than 100 pounds. I remember being ashamed when the picture was shot – after all, every other girl on the beach had abs of steel while my belly rounded to the barest possible little pouch. My visual treat count was not at a hundred percent. And it never would be, because no number on the scale, no reflection in the mirror, was ever enough.

I could never really believe I was attractive at all. Case in point:

At a wedding reception, I went to the bar to ask the bartender for a drink. He looked at me intently and said: "Well, *hi*. Where have you been all day?"

I was utterly perplexed. What did he care where I had been? I settled on saying "Sitting over there in a chair," and returned to my friends. "The bartender asked me a very strange question," I said. "Why did he want to know what chair I'd been sitting in?"

They fell on the floor laughing. "Mickie, that was a *line*; he was *flirting* with you," they said.

To me, being flirted with simply wasn't an option. I assumed that was reserved for other, more acceptable girls – girls who were thinner, better dressed or richer, more confident and comfortable with boys. Doubtless there were males who genuinely flirted with me, thousands of them for all that I knew. But if so I they probably thought I was rejecting them. In fact I just hadn't recognized the signs. I could have been a heartbreaker, and I wouldn't have had a clue.

During a job interview for a teaching position the school superintendent said, "It's great to be so young and pretty, but how are you going to deal with all the boys falling in love with you?" I literally turned around to see who he was talking to.

When my son was quite young, we were walking down a fairway where the "carnies" ran games. As we passed by, one of the carnies addressed us both. "Um-uh," he said. "If I had a mother that looked like that, I'd have never left home."

It was better than being called "wide load." But I was equal parts pleased and extremely freaked out. Contrary to my father's ideas, (which I have absorbed whether I wanted to or not) I didn't want to be a walking entertainment or freak show. I didn't ask for anything that day except being David's mother and having fun at the fair. The carnies' comment didn't feel complimentary; it felt more like verbal rape.

I wanted to be pretty, but I was scared to be pretty. During my slimmer incarnations I dressed to look as sexy and desirable as possible. I wanted everyone who saw me to *think* I was sexy and desirable. It made me feel powerful.

But when a man in K-Mart siddled up to me and whispered "You're sexy" in my ear I panicked. It scared me – I wanted to be admired, not someone's "Blue Light Special". I wanted to say, "Thanks Buddy" and "Leave me alone!" at the same time. He had violated the rules I had made to keep myself safe. These were: look, be impressed, don't touch, and shut up.

THE MYSTERY THAT BINDS ME STILL

In fact, I had all the symptoms of sexual molestation, which puzzled me. Because I haven't been molested.

But I had had the "bladder stretching" treatments and, to my surprise, according to a sexual abuse counselor, that rated as sexual abuse. It had many of the features of rape – it was done against my will, it hurt, and a man was shoving something tubular-shaped through my private parts. My terror of men, of sex and of being a woman all fit right in with being bi-polar: divided and afraid.

It doesn't help that I live in a culture so conflicting in its messages. Am I supposed to be Marilyn Monroe or Twiggy? Anna Nichole or Kate Moss? Put false things on my body or take false things off? Hack up my face, have breast reduction, put in silicone implants, smash my breasts down in a "minimizer" or haul 'em up in a wonder bra?

In middle age, I face other challenges as well. All the ladies on television tell me I must dye my gray hair, smear my face with "anti-aging" creams, inject my wrinkled areas with toxins and deny my age.

I walk into a beauty salon, and the first thing the owner says is, "You must be here to color your hair."

"This *is* my hair color," I say.

"You'd look younger if your hair was dyed," she replies.

"But what do I need to look younger **for?**"

I'm confused and confounded again.

I am traversing the human path of life, which dictates I am to grow and change and age. I've already mutated from child to adolescent, adolescent to young adult, young adult to parenthood, etc. I got my first period and my first hot flashes more or less when I was supposed to. But now that I'm in my fifties, I'm told the whole process has got to stop. I must halt sagging gravity, grab the Botox, tighten my ass, sign up for cosmetic surgery, and for heaven's sake, if I *must age*, do it with a body like Cher's.

But I don't even *want* to look like Cher.

Being gray haired and overweight in America makes me invisible. Sometimes I resent that. Sometimes I'm glad.

The woman whose physical aspect impressed me the most was not featured in a Bowflex commercial. In fact, I met her at Mass at a friend's church. I never spoke with her; I only saw her from behind. She was an older woman who stood in a way I had never seen before, her arms flung out in prayer. I watched her cup her hands as if she was inviting Spirit into her soul, her whole body embracing the air.

I had just had my baby. I was scared and anxious and insecure. Sudden motherhood was terrifying. I wondered if I'd be up to it at all.

The woman's wrinkled arms stretched forth to her Lord. Suddenly, I wondered how many children had been held in those arms, how many nights she had spent sitting up with a sick child. I wanted her to tell me all about life, what I could expect and what I should avoid. I wondered if she could teach me to capture joy as she did, to abandon my arms to celebration in the air. Speechlessly, powerfully, she had led me into faith. For that moment, I believed I'd have the strength to take whatever comes.

Now that was a beautiful woman.

Mickie R. Singer

CHAPTER ELEVEN – TEACHER: REBEL WITH A CAUSE

The Teacher's College I attended was in danger of losing its accreditation. The reasons for this were obvious. They barely touched on curriculum, lesson plans, units, and grading; their idea of teaching me discipline was to ask what I'd do if a student of mine got icing on a map from an illegally eaten cinnamon bun. Square on Madagascar, I believe it was.

My answer was simple. "I'd lick it off."

I would have too, but unfortunately real discipline problems were no so easily disposed. For example, no one had prepared me for Dader Junior High, and Ronald Hall.

On a breezy September day it was my first time as a fulltime teacher. My 7th grade English class was all seated in their appointed rows. I put my head down – just for a moment – checking attendance in the manner we educators refer to as "taking role."

Kelly Highman in a back row seat called in a high, piercing voice: "Miss Singer! Ronald Hall just jumped out of the window!"

Indeed he had. He was halfway across the meadow by the time I saw where he'd gone. We were on the first floor, so he'd come to no harm. He was clearly a man of action, and would give me other opportunities to admire his direct, take-charge style.

Things went both uphill – and downhill - from there.

THE MYSTERY THAT BINDS ME STILL

I was barely 22 when I began teaching. I had no idea how to handle the kids at Dader, all of whom were brimming with hormones, largely hostile, and taller than I was. Out of all of them, I ended up liking window-diver Ronald Hall the best. He amused me. Whenever I'd keep him after school for detention – which was often – he'd surround me in a circle waving his fists. "I'm gonna fight you, Miss Singer," he'd tell me. "I'm gonna fight you." But he never did.

It was a horrible first year. My friend and mentor, Lorraine Kappell, told me to put my feet on the classroom floor and stay there, which is about all I did. One of the few amusing memories I have of Dader was the girl in my class who gave the plural of "grass" as "lawn."

Luckily, my feet were able to stick on the floor through the year, long enough to be blessedly transferred to a high school the following year. High school was where I wanted to be anyway. There's a world of difference between the hormonal raging of younger and older adolescents. Fourteen year olds look at a wall and bounce off of it. Fifteen year olds look at a wall and wonder why they have to be inside of it. I can handle that.

When I moved on to high school I felt more at home – especially since it was one of the high schools I had attended. It was the second and third year of my teaching career, which means I was still trying to learn how I'd be the teacher I wanted to be. I was such a creampuff and I knew it, so I picked some iron-clad rule, just to make the students think I was tough. The first couple of years I refused to let them chew gum in class. The truth is I could have cared less if they chewed it. I just wanted them to think I did. It worked. One of my colleagues told me she'd overheard one of my students in her study hall. "That Miss Singer, she's strict," the girl claimed. "She won't even let you chew gum."

My greatest discovery was in realizing I didn't have to act like a bitch.

Back, when I was in college – and sadly, still today, aspiring teachers are told to be in rigid control of their classes. The classic line is "don't smile until Christmas."

With a few exceptions my high school teachers had been boring, demanding and largely mean. They taught content, not students. Everything came from textbooks and worksheets. Asking questions was not valued; unquestioning obedience was. I wanted to do it differently.

I remember one teacher whose creative lesson plan was to "have students experience muscular response." To this end, she had situated a thumbtack, nail side up, on everyone's seat. Luckily on that day Jody and I came early and discovered them so we removed the tacks before the students could sit on them. The teacher bitterly complained.

I had to learn how to balance the rebellious student I had been with what was realistically required of me now. I had to draw the perimeters – particularly by learning what perimeters worked for me. Seating students rigidly in rows and lecturing to them from notes were not successful methods for me. Doing what I could to bring them firsthand to understand learning – and *what* they were learning – were my perimeters, and the boundary lines shifted from time to time – depending on the students, depending on my mood, depending on the weather outside or the hour of the day. One thing I learned in teaching was I had to go with the flow. In educator language it's called "monitor and adjust." When the situation is hopeless, it's "let this be a challenge to you."

One of my priorities was that I didn't want the students to be bored. I knew that when I got bored I didn't learn. I also found that when I got bored it was hard to teach.

It followed that I made efforts to create lessons – and a way of teaching them – that wouldn't be boring. Not all of the efforts took, but I tried. I regard teaching as my most glorious experience. I can't imagine having a job more enjoyable, more challenging and stressful, more delightful or more memorable. I loved it, every hideous and happy moment. Nothing was predictable, no expectation fulfilled precisely as I thought it would. The kids were annoying, horrible, immensely lovable and the light of my life. They touched and moved me in ways I never thought possible; they made me laugh and Lord, how they made me cry.

I never did learn how to teach. Things changed from year to year. The kids did, the administration did, and I did. What worked wonderfully one year, or even in one class, didn't always work the next year or in the next class. I was constantly learning from them, constantly trying to find ways to make them understand that what they were learning was real and mattered to their lives. Sometimes it worked.

Teachers are taught to control their classes, yet the irony is the kids, no matter how obedient, are never under control. It is not the teenagers' nature. It *is* their nature to discover, to challenge, to push the envelope. Poised in their nether-world of neither child nor adult, self-control is not at the top of their list.

I considered myself a role model, although some of my co-workers would strongly disagree. I let students know growing up was nothing to be afraid of; that you could be an adult and still have fun, and that amusement doesn't need to come from "blowing weed" or haunting bars. I believed in being a teacher in the fullest sense - not just subject and content but of them, the experience of being human, and their lives.

In the classroom I had beanbag chairs and pillows; they could use them or lay on the floor. My experience was that it didn't close their minds to escape their desks, it opened them more. I decorated the room with bright splashes of color: kites, stars and wind chimes hanging from the ceiling, knots of colored silks across the walls. I had two mannequins, female and male, which they named Woodrow and Matilda. They made for a great opening gambit. Inevitably the kids would ask why I had mannequins in the room. I'd tell

THE MYSTERY THAT BINDS ME STILL

them I had no idea; they must supply the answer. Thus the yearly first writing assignment was born.

I also had a silk flower garden with a sundial, a birdbath and a gnome – a homemade fountain (which the kids filled with a goldfish they called James and took responsibility for feeding) odd hats, snippets of poetry, anything I could find that fit into my concept of "the attic of the mind." I wanted the students stimulated. The environment worked. It was both comfortable and challenging. At any rate, *I liked it.*

In all my years of teaching, there is one thing I am proudest of. I had a tough class and couldn't find a way to deal with them at all. They were a group of loud, aggressive boys who didn't like me one bit and let me know it. The hostility between us grew until I thought they, me, or the class would explode. One Monday I announced that we were going to talk. They were free to tell me what they thought of me and why and I would do the same in return. I asked for absolute honesty. I also told them we were going to work this out if it took all week long.

It did. I took an earful. In turn I told them how I felt. By Friday, we were alright. The greatest blessing for me in this experience was I got to know the kids. Instead of the arrogant, hostile front they'd presented, I learned lots of good stuff about them. The student who I felt had disliked me the most – and given me the hardest time – turned out to be a kid with a heck of a soft side. I even got to learn more about him from his Mom. .

Mickie R. Singer

Being bi-polar my moods went up and down in the classroom as well. When I was depressed I mostly hid it, but wasn't always successful. The last thing I wanted to do was go into a rage. I practiced being soft-voiced and patient, taking breaths and counting to ten, being as gentle as I could. If I had a discipline problem I usually took the student out in the hall and talked with him/her as quietly as I could. I was pretty good at this; a student said to me once, "How come you put up with us and all the other teachers yell at us?" But sure enough – to my shame – there were times when I got overwhelmed, and a couple of times, the rage did get aimed at a student. It happened very rarely, but I deeply regret that it ever happened at all.

I had relatively few problems with discipline. This was not because I was strong in the disciplinary area; quite the opposite. I clearly sent the message that I was the head of the classroom and what I would say would go; I didn't let any of them step on me or treat me with disrespect. But when it came down to trying to be fierce or mean or demanding – forget it. I couldn't get away with it, didn't want to do it to begin with, and early in my teaching years learned that that stance wasn't for me. One of my students teased me by naming me "The Great Intimidator." My main disciplinary method was to threaten to put a peach pit up their nose. Before our schools were thrown into the crucible of sexual harassment charges/ political correctness, I would also threaten to come over and sit on a child's head; at one point I told a male student that if he didn't shut up I was going to come over there and kiss him. He shut up immediately, while another student observed "My, I don't think I've ever heard a teacher take that approach before."

In many of my job interviews I had, I encountered a curious attitude, which was expressed in a variety of forms. But it always came down to: "You're so short, how can you teach?" I found it astonishing that anyone would think that height, or weight, or the ability to intimidate had anything to do with how a teacher was capable to teach. Walking the halls at Woodward High School I once saw a six foot male teacher being bodily removed from his class. In my recent years in the faculty room I was amused to hear male faculty members complain that now that corporeal punishment was no longer allowed they could no longer control their students by a swift smack in the head. These were attitudes of the same ilk I had found as a student. To be effective teachers had to be bullies and students were fair game. Not in my classroom, thank you.

I didn't want to give my students the old traditional writing assignments so I tried something new. Where I was teaching most of the kids were white. I contacted a teacher at a school where most of the kids were black, and we set up a pen pal program. Not only did the kids write back and forth, but we also visited each other's classes in our respective schools. It was an eye-opening experience all around. I'll never forget one flustered female student of mine who was bewildered about how to communicate with her flirtatious pen pal, a black male.

"He wrote that he's built like Wesley Snipes," she said. "What should I write back?"

I told her to tell him she was built like Wesley Snipes, too.

I got into trouble doing one of my most effective lessons of all. I had done it for years and it always made a memorable point. It was designed to get kids thinking about what the process of learning is about. The principal walked in to observe me at the beginning of class. I – fat dumb and happy – thought he was just going to *love* it.

I began by asking them if they'd ever observed a two-year old out for a walk. We talked about how different the child's reaction is to the world – unlike us he takes nothing for granted; he is fascinated with all he surveys. I asked them if they remembered how they behaved in elementary school. When a teacher asked a question, many of their arms went eagerly up. Now no one wants to answer questions in the classroom at all. What happened, I asked them. What was so different now?

Then I took out a jar of applesauce, dipped into its contents, and smeared it all over my face, in my nose and on my hair. "What do I look like?" I'd say.

"Like a little kid playing with his food," they'd answer.

Right. "What does a little kid's face look like when he does this?" They'd tell me he would have a big smile on his face. I asked them to think about why. Did he know he was getting away with something socially acceptable? Was mischief his goal?

Eventually they'd get to where I was guiding them to go. The answer was the kid smiles because he is happy doing what he's doing – and what he is doing is *learning.*

I'd announce that today they would re-experience what they used to know, that learning is not drudgery. To do this I put several teaspoons of applesauce on everyone's desks along with a small paper cup of water and a stack of paper towels. Their instructions were to play with the applesauce; the only rules being the applesauce must stay on their desks or on their persons and nowhere else.

After a bit we'd clean up and I'd ask them what they learned. They had all kinds of discoveries. Applesauce was very grainy; it was cold even when it wasn't refrigerated; it had a peculiar smell, it could be used like finger-paint, it was sticky and hard to clean up. We ended by talking about the process we had been through, what it involved and how we responded to it. I used it as an opportunity to talk about the importance of curiosity. Through the years students let me know how memorable that lesson was for them. Their younger siblings and classmates wanted to get into my class so they could experience it. I thought it was pretty good.

The next day I was called to the principal's office. When I walked in he went berserk. He threatened to fire me. He said what I'd done was "out there" in the community. He said I'd better be careful, that I had a target on my back, and that I drove the older teachers crazy. I was forbidden to *ever* do the applesauce lesson again.

Gradually, I was "forbidden" to do more and more things. One day before Easter holiday I conducted a two-minute egg hunt. Afterwards I was called to the principal's office.

"Miss Singer," he said, "I need you to explain to me how an Easter egg hunt fits into the English curriculum." Someone had ratted on me. I was furious, and I had had it. "It doesn't have a damn thing to do with it," I told him. "People around here have got to CHILL OUT."

An incident that tore my heart out was the day I answered a loud knock after school on my door. There stood a kid I barely knew, surrounded by his friends who were laughing at him. "Let me in, please, lady," the kid said. "I gotta talk to you."

He slipped inside and stood against the wall, suddenly bawling. This kid had a reputation of being an extremely tough kid. What he said next was probably the toughest thing he ever did.

"I gotta tell somebody," he cried. "I never told anybody. I'm gonna tell you. My father has been raping me for years."

I was mandated to call the Victim Center and that's exactly what I did. I stayed with him, and then took him back to a friend's house, giving him my phone number and telling him to feel free to call. On Monday I realized I'd have to let him know I had to break his confidence. He'd begged me not to tell anyone, but I had to report any abuse. I asked the probation officer to help me explain it. It didn't go well. The young man quit school and I never saw him again.

I also have gobs of fond memories, all the myriad of happy moments with the kids. The student who played "drums" on his desk until I drummed at him back; the school-wide game of tag we played - initiated by me tapping a student and telling her she was "it" – the day the mannequins got married, and all the classes held their own weddings, with DJ's and written vows and the "bride" and "groom" decked out in proper wedding dress. The day I fell asleep during Reading Day. I had a nightmare, and screamed. Talk about finding ways to get the attention of the class.

There was the girl who never smiled until one day in class I said I wished she would, and she was smiling and chatty ever since. The student whose final exam made me laugh for days; she wrote that she was astonished that "Anne Frank could live so long without food or water or air." It astonished me, as well. And the boy who had thought about suicide years ago who told me he was doing okay – and that I'd made a difference – when he'd returned after senior year to the prom.

What I enjoyed the most – and what equally alarmed me – was that I never knew what was going to happen next. Part of that was me with my capricious mouth. Words were always coming out before I thought better than to say them. During a lesson in diversity, I asked two kids to "fill in the blanks" with the first words that came to their minds. I had just begun listing them: Whites are....Blacks   always....Jews have.....Homosexuals are..." when Lenny, well-known as a homophobic, shouted out: "I hate *fags*! They all play with themselves!"

The Fastest Mouth in the West opened up. "And you *don't*?" I said.

It is not wise to publicly accuse your student of masturbating, and not at all recommended in the Curriculum guide, but it got Lenny to shut up. The class rose in unison to give me a standing ovation.

If the kids remained silent too long after I'd asked a question I'd threaten to sing Broadway show tunes - badly. Then I'd do it. I quit when I caught on they were so amused by this that they were purposely playing dumb.

In 2000 I resigned. If I hadn't I would have lost my spirit – and my mental health. The kids were great, but trying to fit in into a school community where I was the proverbial square peg in a round hole exacted a payment that, after ten years, I could no longer afford. I was sick way too much of the time, even hospitalized with stomach pain as a result of stress. Working surrounded by disapproval was like being back at Bond Hill, so queer again. In every which way there was, it hurt.

The principal had already let me know there was a good possibility I'd have a bad evaluation at the end of the year. They were less and less enthused about the nature of my lessons and my independent attitude. It was clear to me they wanted me to go.

I left regretting, lost and not knowing what to do next. If I wasn't going to teach, what would I do? If I wasn't going to be a teacher, what could I be? For most of my adult life, a teacher was what I was and what I had always wanted to be. I couldn't conceive of myself as anything else. It was like losing my heart.

I still get hungry for the smell of chalk and markers, the scent of cafeteria food, hallways scattered with paper airplanes, water fountains jammed with gum. School is a world unlike anything else. Looking back at how I hated it when I was a kid, who would have guessed I'd never want to leave?

CHAPTER TWELVE – MY PRINCE, AT LAST

As a little girl, I would lie in bed and fantasize about my prince – the man who would love, rescue and marry me - what he would be like, what he would do. For no discernible reason, I was sure his name was going to be Peter. He would appear from the trees, like some fairytale Tarzan, and fill my heart completely evermore.

No one named Peter ever arrived. Not even Peter Pan.

As I got older my needs for a prince changed. Priority one was that he had to accept a crazy woman who trembled upon occasion and threw up. How this was ever going to happen, I hadn't a clue.

However, my 22nd birthday was marked by two momentous events. One was an extraordinary cake made by my friend Susan. The other was the soon-to-be-coming of my prince.

Cincinnati is a city of hills, lots of them. Stand on top of any of them, chances are you'll be rewarded with an unforgettable view. Such was the case looking down a particular hill in the wintertime. Through the leafless trees at night one could see a pattern of streetlights – which clearly spelled out the word "SHIT."

I was quite enamored of this view and took lots of people up the hill to see it. When Susan baked me a birthday cake, she personalized it using little plastic gnomes to celebrate my magical nature. There were twenty-two of them stuck into the icing, in a pattern that spelled out "SHIT."

THE MYSTERY THAT BINDS ME STILL

Looking back, that was my metaphor for what came next. It seemed so sweet and witty and delicious, who would have thought it would turn bitter? The prince, of course – not the cake.

I began teaching at age 21; sure I was headed for the traditional schoolmarm spinsterhood. This thought came from my zero-Fahrenheit self-esteem. In all things, particularly in my potential for romantic relationships, I feared I was invisible. I had always felt invisible inside my family (my father once introduced "all his children" –while all three of us were clearly standing in the room – as "Barry and Jon." It was quite disheartening.)

I dealt with it by becoming Ms. Jekyl/Ms. Hyde. On one hand, I didn't even exist; on the other I kept my presence, my opinions and my voice as loudly apparent as I could at all times – just so I could be seen at all. It was not a formula for believing I could be loved, much less for success.

By age 22, the most successful relationship I had had was my catch-as-can with Traveler, who had told me he loved me when he walked out the door. It did not bode well for the future.

But things changed when my friend Jody introduced me to a man who had moved next door. He was in radio, my students' favorite station, in fact. Barely beginning my teaching career, I was being cursed with recurring laryngitis. He seemed to be the perfect answer for me, a guest speaker for my tenth grade English class.

I didn't know him very well. The few times I had bumped into him at Jody's I had the impression he was a bit of a bumpkin. He rarely opened his mouth and when he did it was only to ask questions. I thought that was a sign he wasn't very bright.

As I listened to him speak in the classroom, I felt like Paul riding his donkey on the way to Damascus – I saw the light and was knocked off my ass. He was obviously not just bright but extremely so. He was confident and open and good-humored. He talked to the kids with such ease; it was as if he had taught in a classroom all his life. This man, I thought, was a "*mensch*."

"*Mensch*" is a Yiddish word which directly translated simply means "person." But the connotation of it is much more. A "*mensch*" is someone with fire and guts and courage, who has come into his own. A "*mensch*" is genuine and honest and real. A "*mensch*" has *chutzpah* (balls).

I was fascinated by his self-possession, his gentleness, his sense of humor and his sweet smile. I asked him if I could do anything to thank him and to my relief and joy he asked me out.

I found he was all the things I wanted and more. He had genuine charm, a center of goodness that radiated from him. He was wonderfully whimsical, funny, thoughtful and sensitive. He liked earthy women, like me. He was not carved out of any restrictive box and wasn't interested in anyone who was. He was tolerant and supportive and *accepting* most of all.

THE MYSTERY THAT BINDS ME STILL

Shortly after we began dating he witnessed one of my attacks. I had to leave right in the middle of a movie. We sat on Fountain Square, his arm around me while I hyperventilated and shook. *And he didn't go away.* He came right back to me the next day.

It was then that he became the prince.

There was only one problem – he smoked marijuana, usually every day. I have had my fill of that. I told him point blank, it's either me or the drugs.

He chose me, of course. I never gave a thought to the bottles of vodka he began buying. He combined the stuff with red Hawaiian punch, a more noxious concoction I cannot conceive. *That* should have told me something right away.

He was a wonderful playmate, and a cooperative one. He put up with pretending to be Frankie Avalon because I wanted to be Annette Funicello. He bought me an electric train to put under the Christmas tree. We took trips out of the city so I could see what a pumpkin field looked like. He had been raised in rural, woodsy Pennsylvania; my utter city-girl experience amused him. He fascinated me with stories of the Norman Rockwell childhood he had lived back home. On whatever rare occasion in Cincinnati a thing of nature occurred he made sure I saw it. The most impressive was when the Ohio River froze (only the second time in a century): He told me the Susquehanna River, where he lived, froze every year. It was as if, just for me, he'd reinvented the wheel.

He laughed at me and with me; he seemed to find everything I did amusing or charming in some way. Most of all, he loved that I ran to kiss him when he walked in the door, and I loved that he loved it. He was more than my prince. I made him a god.

It must have been quite a burden for him. Whatever he said was right, and the truth. He said so, and I believed it. I asked him everything and he gave me the answers, down to whether I should take aspirin for a headache. It was wonderful to surrender my self-ness to him, wonderful to be taken care of. I needed him deeply and he knew it. He loved that, too.

We were, in short, the classic flamingly codependent couple. I was terrified he'd leave me; so I'd keep my mouth shut and seldom disagreed argue with him. I didn't ask for respect; while he demanded respect. He was insecure, too, and afraid of my leaving *him*. So he always kept me at just a little distance, to keep me unsteady on my feet. When he told me I did something wrong I would stay silent and hang my head in shame, as if I were a child.

I was easily manipulated. All he had to do was tell me how pretty his former girlfriend was – which he did often – and I'd fold. I adopted her as my own personal ghost to whom I would never measure up.

Yet with whatever was bad there was much that was good. We loved the hell out of each other. For a long time we functioned as a team.

THE MYSTERY THAT BINDS ME STILL

My prince was my best friend whom I trusted utterly. I felt that he accepted everything about me and I was grateful for what I considered a tall order. I had no idea that the night I had my first anxiety attack in front of him, he actually thought I was crazy. Later he told me he found me "intriguing" enough that he hung on.

So when he began berating me for not folding the sandwich meat correctly or hanging the washrags right, I assumed I deserved it. His derision for my "failings" combined with protestations of his love was familiar to me. It was my family all over again. I slipped into my old familiar "bad girl" position and fit right into the mold.

The shift in our relationship began when he started suffering from untreated depression and abusing valium. I didn't recognize he had a problem; I knew nothing, at the time, about depression, and after all, valium was a prescription drug. Gradually, though, the prince changed. Between the valium and the depression he became distant and withdrawn. He slept all the time and when he didn't I wished he would because he was getting very mean.

I had had very few boyfriends and even fewer experiences; when the prince came along I glommed onto his side like a barnacle to a ship. Even though not once in four years had he told me he loved me, I bought a house with him and waited for him to say it. I was completely dependent on him; he was my rock. Without him, I would sink. It was necessary to trust him utterly, and I did. Even though I was embarrassed to be living together and hurt that he hadn't asked me to marry him, I shoved it aside –after all, I "wasn't good enough." It all fit the mold.

It took four years for the prince to propose. He turned to me one day and said, "Alright, I'm tired of listening to you bitch. Set the date."

It never occurred to me that his proposal was neither romantic, loving, respectful – nor that it was downright insulting. I truly didn't know I deserved better. Yet things were to get much, much worse.

I had known all along that the prince could be controlling. As tolerant and sweet as he could be, he could turn around and be just as critical and mean. But the first seven years I was with him, his nature was a lot sweeter and a lot less mean. Seven years is a long time to know a person; it was too much of a shock to see that he wasn't that person anymore. I went into denial, big time.

When our marriage began its downward spin, the prince began making nasty remarks. Here's a brief selection: "For God's sake, why don't you put your things in a briefcase? You look like a damn bad lady, toting things around in a sack." or "Why'd you leave this pot soaking in the sink? Don't you have any idea of how to care for your things?" or "An idiot wouldn't have burnt that soup. How could you be so stupid?"

His parents were there The Night I Burnt The Soup. They found it amusing. He found it unforgivable.

THE MYSTERY THAT BINDS ME STILL

His comments were usually designed to blindside me. I had no idea when they would come, and they seldom came when I would expect it. For no discernible reason I heard them when I stepped out the door, or picked a toy up from the carpet or made a meal – in short, at any time during the course of everyday life. This was a very clever maneuver on his part – it kept me off-balanced, confused and waiting for the other shoe to drop.

I began to look for ways I could escape while still with David and in reach of the house. One year I planted a small garden and that sucker was as weeded as a garden could be. Every night I'd be out there, pulling weeds, imaginary and otherwise. I found the smell of earth to be tranquilizing, as I also did hot baths. I probably held the world's record for refilling hot water and laying in the tub. Away from the prince.

I am far from a stupid person, yet I couldn't get it into my head that the prince was dead. A number of dragons had slain him. I kept hanging on wanting to believe in his resurrection, my sweet kind prince who would come again.

As he and we began to change, the line between us was erased. In his mind, I was a compendium of him. I was expected to comport myself as he would, and since that was beyond me, he could offer up an endless series of complaints. Even my body was not allowed to be separate from his. When I tried a new hair style that involved getting my hair cut he accused me of doing it to spite him and wouldn't speak to me for days. I wept with guilt. It never occurred to me that it was my right to cut my own hair.

He was angry and threatened by what meant the most to me, especially if it was different from his view of things. "I want you to stop going to Al-Anon, I want you to stop going to therapy, and I don't want you to keep doing your storytelling. I want you to do these three things for me," he'd say." It isn't asking much."

He might as well have asked that I remove twenty buckets of blood. He never heard me tell a story. When I joined Al-Anon, he all but went through the roof.

One Thanksgiving I cooked him a turkey even though we'd already been to dinner at his sister's house. Since there'd be no leftovers, I wanted to provide the prince with some more turkey to eat. When I set it on the table he saw I had forgotten to take the giblets out. The package was still stuffed in the cavity. "That's it," he said. He packed his suitcase and left the house. He didn't call. He didn't come back until late the next day.

I had developed a problem in my legs, which later on would include my back. It was painful and sometimes kept me from walking. In the early years, my legs had once collapsed. The prince picked me up and carried me through the streets. (A very prince-like act, indeed.) But years later, when we visited my folks in Cincinnati, he drew me into a bedroom and berated me, fiercely: "We just can't do anything together anymore, and it's all because of you. You used to look good and

THE MYSTERY THAT BINDS ME STILL

I was proud to be with you. Now you're fat and your face is always pale. You put on make-up but it looks horrible. Why can't you be like other women and know how to make-up on right? And what's worse," he went on, "we used to be able to take walks. *Now you can't walk.*"

It was the nastiest, most shaming thing he ever said. In many ways he was correct. I felt crippled in every way I could be.

One night he had given me rare "permission" to celebrate a happy occasion with some friends. He was invited, but refused to come along. He knew we were going to a "golden oldies place" to dance. The club closed at 2 a.m., which is when I came home. The next morning he ordered me to sit at the table while he had his say. "You've gone too far, Mickie," he said. "This time you've gone too far. Just what do you mean by being out without me AFTER MIDNIGHT?"

I had no idea that being out past this time I had committed a marital crime, but he was furious. So much so that I immediately began to feel I had done something terribly wrong. The only thing that stopped his tirade was a phone call bringing the news that his father had suffered a heart attack.

That shut him up – for a while.

When I became pregnant his anger came to a head. Instead of being supportive he called me "Orca" and the "Great Whale." He made innumerable comments about how I took naps and moved slowly, whereas the pregnant women he worked with were full of energy. (In fact, I had gestational diabetes at the time, which neither of us knew). When the doctor told me I couldn't lift very much he refused to help with the groceries. Instead I had to hire a kid in the neighborhood to go with me and carry the food into the house. It didn't occur to me that he really should have lent a hand.

He came to Lamaze classes, which I felt was supportive, until he told me he just didn't see how I was going to make it through birth.

I knew life with the prince had become hell but I had no idea I was actually putting up with abuse. I thought abuse was only when somebody hit you and the prince was way too smart to even think of even doing that to me. Touch me and Mack Singer's daughter would have come out fighting; that was the one thing that would have set me off. But he didn't need fists with me – his words were the weapons.

It didn't occur to me to leave him, either. After years of being told how worthless I was I truly believed it. His strategy was to confront me with all the ways I was ruining his life. Except for when I went into the psych ward, I had never felt so "all gone."

It was hard to recognize myself, hard to hold onto being a real grownup person who had the right to make choices and be treated with respect. Except in the outside world I had ceased to know that I was an adult with rights.

I was living with someone who terrified me. I'd have gone through ten psych ward lockups rather than go through the horror of that. I had no rest from fear except for where I could still

THE MYSTERY THAT BINDS ME STILL

function, in my friendships and in my job. At home I barely existed. My main activity was lowering my head in shame. I felt and acted like a whipped puppy – slinking around, waiting for the next blow to come.

Only a few people outside our closed door had any idea of what really went on inside of it. I didn't have any bruises on my body to show. My vulnerability was inside, where my soul was crushed. It's possible that I would have left sooner if I had realized that I qualified for an abused woman's shelter. Today mental and emotional abuse is considered powerful stuff. The only criterion to enter our local shelter now is that a woman feels afraid.

Being with the prince was like living with someone who dwelled underwater. Every once in a while he would emerge – the old he, the prince that I loved. And then my heart would tug and I'd be good for hanging in there again, denial coming on strong.

I was, as in the Julia Roberts movie, "sleeping with the enemy." Accepting that he was no longer my prince was the realization hardest and longest to come to. Getting out of there, in comparison, was relatively quick.

The benchmark was when the prince went to one of his occasional forays into therapy (he'd stick with it for about two months and then fire the therapist). After a few sessions the new therapist asked me to come in too. I was surprised and alarmed. Could this mean there was something wrong with my marriage?

Duh.

The day before our second session I was reading Ann Lander's column. In it was a letter from a woman who wrote that she believed she had become an "enabler." What she described, in response to her husband's alcoholism, sounded eerily close to my behavior in regard to the drug use of my prince. Likely, he always sent me to buy his pills. And I was the one who called his work to say he was sick when he was really just zombie out. I said as much in the therapy session. "I think I'm an enabler."

"Bingo!" replied the therapist. "You are, and your husband is a drug addict."

The prince literally sat there and just grinned.

I figured if I was an enabler I'd better learn not to be. The next day I walked into an Al-Anon meeting and suddenly found myself feeling very much at home. It was as if I spoke Martian all my life and suddenly I had discovered a whole group of people who spoke Martian too.

It was a while before I understood that codependent behavior was codependent behavior; it doesn't matter what the impetus is. My mood for the day depended on how my prince was. He was chugging valium, but I was getting sicker yet. It was all very familiar again – alcoholism and other such addictions become a family disease, because everyone's behavior changes in sick ways in response to the loved one's illness. Years later I recognized why I was so at home in Al-Anon. Mental illness is a family illness, too, with many of the same symptoms as a family touched by alcoholism. Having a mentally ill parent, I needed to be in control, needed to be a caretaker, never knew what to expect, learned to keep family secrets – the whole nine yards. I had practiced to perfection taking on somebody else's life to save my own.

I was in Al-Anon, going to several meetings a week for five years, before I finally became strong enough to reclaim who I was. Part of what made Al-Anon so powerful was the understanding and support of the people in the groups. I could (and at times did) call people in the middle of the night; one fellow member arrived at my door to comfort me at 4 a.m. They understood when, on occasions, I had irrational fear of the prince. They would answer my phone calls at 3:30 p.m. because that's when I'd start to get nervous – the prince would soon be coming home.

I felt boxed in and he had all the controls. I was in Al-Anon and in therapy, yet I still felt unable to get out. Even when my parents came to visit and saw how it was I didn't believe they could help. Typically of an abused spouse, I believed myself beyond assistance.

I didn't dare think of leaving and on the rare occasions I did I couldn't imagine any place to go. The prince often told me how hard I was to live with. It was incredibly healing when I asked an Al-Anon member if she thought she could live with me. She paused and thought about it – *really thought about it* – and told me she believed she could. It gave me hope.

Al-Anon encouraged detachment - loving detachment if possible, but detachment. I couldn't imagine detaching from the prince. I couldn't conceive of doing anything he wouldn't like. But one night I asked if he wanted to go to a campfire program. He refused. I asked if he'd mind if I took our son. He didn't say no, but he expressed his derision and scorn. My desire to do it disappeared like air out of a balloon – which, of course, was his intent. But something in me rallied and I did it anyway. I felt a little shaky, but I told myself we'd all survive and there was nothing wrong in doing what I did. I had detached.

My second detachment came when I returned home from a very rare weekend away. I'd performed storytelling in concert at a university. It had been wonderful, and I was flying high. The prince noticed this and saw his opportunity to punish me for what I had done. He asked if I would like for us to order subs and I joyfully agreed. When we sat at the table and unrolled them onto our plates, he said: "I can't imagine how you can let yourself eat that. Look at you. You're fat as a pig, and you're going to eat a sub."

My prince had spoken. For years, I had given him charge of me, including my physical self. It was his right to judge me and more importantly it was his right to keep me in line – *especially* when it came to food. We both knew in that area I had no control. He was just trying to rescue me from myself.....I didn't take a bite of my sub.

THE MYSTERY THAT BINDS ME STILL

Suddenly I realized what was really going on. He wasn't concerned about my health or even my looks – this was just another way he tried to keep me under his control! I happily ate the whole sub.

My final detachment, like all the other things, came gradually. Christmas that year was horrible. The prince lost his temper with me and our son, threw the tree on the floor, and didn't come out of his room for several days. When he came out he wanted us to play as a family with the electric train. We were supposed to act like nothing had occurred. It was crazy-making. He always contended there was nothing wrong. Even presented with his addiction, he'd just shrug his shoulders and say "Everyone's addicted to something."

I knew that was the last Christmas I would live like that. I knew it – but had no idea how I would insure it.

When I had storytelling work to do he refused to take care of our son, so I would either have to drive him to a babysitter's house or take the babysitter to our house, with the prince right there. That was downright weird. He agreed to celebrate our tenth anniversary by inviting friends for dinner. It ended up that I made beef stroganoff and had dinner with the friends without him. He went to bed before they came and never emerged.

In the spring the prince went on a business trip and invited me and our son to go along. But our son and I were already committed to be in a show and if we ditched it that would be problematical for a lot of people and our son would have been very disappointed. So I told him we couldn't go. This was a major rebellion on my part and it was not well received. When he returned he didn't talk to me for several months. He'd grunt and say hello and that was about the shape of it. He slept all the time and on the rare occasions he was awake I'd pray he'd go back to sleep. Anytime he was awake he was trouble. If I approached him about our difficulties he'd just say he believed in us and everything would be fine. It was a sweet sentiment, and at one time I would have agreed. By that point, however, all I could think was what house was *he* living in?

Yet I still loved the prince. I loved him for who he had once been, who at times he could still be, for the hope that he'd come back to me again. One day I looked at him and had the thought that if I waited for the day that I no longer loved him I would never go. I had to love him but leave. I had to get our son out of that poisonous atmosphere and I had to get myself and my life back. He was unwilling to try to make it better: he had turned down all of my requests to return to therapy, go to marital counseling, or get detoxed at a rehab, which his company would pay for. Every time I thought of the horror of inflicting divorce on our child, I thought of how he might end up losing me, too, because if we didn't leave I would lose my mind.

Two years ago I attended an evening class. A student remarked that she didn't understand why abused women stayed with their abusers.

THE MYSTERY THAT BINDS ME STILL

She said she'd worked with abused women and they were all doormats, and dumb. I politely tried to explain matters to her. But she wouldn't listen; she went back to her original contention. At that point my voice raised several decibels and Mack Singer's daughter was ready to go for her throat. I informed the teacher I would not be able to return; my therapist had suggested I pursue some extracurricular interests for my mental health and the class didn't seem to work.

Some people don't understand the dance of the abused and the abuser, but loosely, this is how it works: Imagine a trauma, any trauma, an accident, a death, a war, a betrayal. The human mind is deeply affected by this kind of stuff. There are results that show up in the victim's thoughts and behavior. They may not seem rational to someone who is not involved. What's rational about losing all trust because one person betrayed you, or refusing to come out in public because you're grieving a death? Stuff happens; we react.

The stuff that happens in abusive situations is insidious. First we're offered love; then we're treated like dirt. I have heard many people contend this sort of thing is cut and dried. They make comments like "If he did that to me I'd be out the door immediately," or "I wouldn't let anyone treat me like that."

Maybe so. But love or believing you are loved is powerful. It's what we all want, wish and hope for. When we think we've got it our grip is usually pretty strong. We'll do an awful lot to hang on. We'll put up with things we wouldn't in anyone but the loved one. We hope that with enough effort, enough faith, we'll make it change back to the way it was.

After a while we'll take responsibility for the whole relationship and if it doesn't get better we'll believe it's our fault. If we are physically, mentally or emotionally abused, or any combination of the three, we begin to believe we are bad. We begin to believe we deserve this abuse. And we see no way out.

Never mind that other people do see ways – never mind that other people don't understand. Within that sad relationship a lot of heavy stuff is going on – manipulation and guilt and being nice one moment and mean the next – it's confusing and conquering and it robs you of yourself. Soon your whole sense of identity is gone.

And we no longer feel safe in our houses or anywhere else because our confidence has been ripped away. We don't believe we'll be taken care of or that we can take care of ourselves. Our self-esteem is in such shreds that we'll cling to the familiar, even if the familiar is awful.

The failure of this marriage is the saddest thing that ever happened to me. All the other things – Mom's mental illness, mine, etc. were awful but I couldn't do anything about them – they were a fact; they were just there. But maybe I could have avoided marrying this person, or left sooner, or been the kind of person who wasn't ripe for feeling bad about me. However, I did the best I could. For those who cannot understand, all I can say is walk a mile in my moccasins and you would.

As in any trauma, the best that can come of it is to learn. And I have. I've made a lot of recovery, I've come a long way, I know now what I'll stand for and what I won't. And I *ain't going back again.*

Being scared of the prince, I was scared of leaving. As it was, I didn't do it alone: I staged an intervention. Earlier in the day I took our son to a friend's house where we were given sanctuary. I returned home. At an appointed time our rabbi and the prince's best friends arrived. Together we all pleaded with the prince to get help. His best friends told him that they had seen him change, that they didn't feel comfortable with our son growing up with him, as he was, in our house. It didn't seem to be getting through. After a few hours I left.

I'd like to say that the prince got help, but he didn't. We got divorced, and the fairytale did not have a happy ending. But I can feel good about one thing: this time, I rescued *myself.*

Cruelly, the prince had once told me I couldn't walk. But I can, right out the door.... Just watch me walk...I can walk, I can walk...

CHAPTER THIRTEEN: LORD, SAVE ME FROM SINGLES DANCES

Once the prince had left the premises, my son David and I returned home. As we came through the door, the house lifted a foot off the ground, moving in a complete 365 degree circle before coming back down. The message was clear: Don't expect this house or your lives to ever be the same again. It's all been turned around.

Of course, the house itself did not speak. It simply created its own little whirlwind, depositing us, unready explorers in the Land of Oz

Believe it – or not.

There was also a great whirling of my head. I fully expected to be married all my life, just like my parents, and for that matter, just like the prince's parents. "Me, Divorced" just wasn't part of my life vocabulary. I wasn't grieving the demise of the marriage because I'd already been doing that for years. I didn't miss the prince. But I was engulfed by anxiety and in its wake, determination. I had no idea how I was going to make this new life work; me a single mother, household breadwinner, mortgage payer, fulltime worker and incompetent maintenance crew for our house. I just knew that I had to do it, so I was going to do it. Few things in my life had ever been as simple and clear.

The entire "how to" came later on.

I had plenty of reassurance from therapist, family and friends. But I knew the most powerful reassurance had to come from me, and that was a hard one to come to. I took to wandering through the house, repeating the refrain of a popular song:

"Somewhere out there
Under the pale moonlight
Someone is thinking of me
And loving me tonight......"

Still, the last thing I wanted at the time was a man. All my energy was going into what I had to do. It would be over six months before I remembered that men were alive, or that I wanted anything to do with them.

Most of all, there was five year old David. I was still working part-time at the paper; what I made there wasn't enough to support both the mortgage and the two of us. I had applied for teaching jobs and blessedly four weeks later a high school job offer came through. David and I just had to hang on until September.

I didn't so much hang on as dig my nails in until I bled. Right after the prince left I had this horrible dream where the garage door was maniacally moving up and down, completely out of my control. It was a highly symbolic dream, but it was a warning too. The house's first temper tantrum was a *disintegrating* garage door. Apparently it was just pasteboard that changed its mind.

There went an immediate drain of several hundred dollars out of my meager savings account. This was to be followed by the brown stain on my T-11 siding disappearing from the outside of the house. Cosmetic needs were not my priority so I let it go until I learned that the stain kept rain and other water from getting into the house. Replacing the garage door had already eaten up my maintenance budget. I was flummoxed until I came up with the answer that would guide me through years of maintenance problems: Competent Friends.

Competent Friends are good-natured people with know-how who are willing to come to things like my staining party, for which they were rewarded with sandwiches and soda and my grateful tears. Among them was Moe who painted and stained houses for a living. He did ¾ of the job himself with the rest pitching in. It was finished in an afternoon.

That taken care of, the next day I came down with mononucleosis. I was all but non-functional for six weeks. Thank God for Sesame Street, friend Norma Ensminger's chicken rice soup and Lyn Buckler from the Jewish Community Center who daily picked David up for camp and delivered him back home. He had to become immersed in television and whatever activities he could find at home. Mommy was broken, and he was on his own.

In fact, David was often on his own. It was all I could do to take charge of daily life and try to stay sane. It was difficult and lonely for David, living with Mommy's bi-polar rages and extreme ups and downs.

At other times, I was a hell of a lot of fun Mom. I let David sleep as often as he liked in a tent we had put up in the living room. We had

THE MYSTERY THAT BINDS ME STILL

impromptu parties for no reason with dinosaur-shaped cakes. When David became curious after seeing a sign announcing an all-night restaurant I woke him after midnight and we went there for hot fudge sundaes. I told him stories and danced for him and sang to him anytime he liked. I took him everywhere I could think of so he could see and learn about anything that caught his interest. I took him along on many of my newspaper assignments. He was treated as royalty by the folks I interviewed, who gave him private showings of plays and concerts and puppet shows. All the neighborhood kids came to our backyard to play softball; I was always a member of the team. Together we played all kinds of things; flying kites, hide and go seek.

I don't anticipate getting any Golden Mom awards. I've had more than my share of parental inadequacies. Nonetheless, I am more at peace with that now. I know – considering everything - I did the best I could.

David is now in his twenties. He has been truly on his own for several years, living elsewhere, paying rent, car insurance and everything else. He's vastly mature and bright, not to mention an extremely good-looking young man. (Masses of dark hair, shoulders like a football player's, big luminous brown eyes). I deeply regret that I often wasn't there for him when he may have needed me most. I know he must have felt lonely and rejected – and unprotected as well. Today, however, he is strong and independent. He follows his own convictions, never swimming with the tide. I like him a lot. He's a mensch.

A few months after our separation, David went to his father for the weekend and I went to a large storytellers' conference. The first night we engaged largely in deep and utter nonsense, putting our cheeks together and communicating through incomprehensible babble. I had a vision of the prince standing above me and saying:" So THIS is it? *This* is why you left me?" In my mind I answered him: "Yup. This is *exactly* why."

My first act of reclamation was to nail green rubber elf shoes to the front door. "There," I thought. "Now anybody who comes to this door is going to know what they'll find behind it. If they don't like it there's no reason for them to come in."

Becoming single again was like walking barefoot in the snow because you lost your shoes. On one hand there was wonderful new freedom; on the other there were disasters that waited to happen and there were no emergency plans in place.

Lightning shut down the well pump twice, the garage door and the air conditioner once. Vast groupings of shingles tore off in heavy winds. I had to put on a whole new roof. The screen door broke, David had croup and needed to go to the doctor but my car wouldn't start, the neighborhood kids threw his shoes in the cornfield and left obscene messages on our answering machine. All spiders and mice within the house I had to kill by myself. I rarely had enough money to take care of these matters, and no source from which I could apply. But we got through it all – with the help of God, miracles, and as always, Competent Friends.

Slowly I grew more confident. I liked my freedom. I felt as if I was getting to know a whole new person, like Pooh who lost his memory one day in the forest. Every time he encountered something he was fond of (like honey) he'd exclaim "So *this* is what Pooh Bear likes!" I was in my own journey of discovery – I was trying new things and revisiting old ones. At each step of the way I could smile and say, "*So this* is what Mickie likes!" I put a new greeting on my answering machine: "Hi, this is Mickie, happy, joyous and free."

Liberation was a-risin' in my breast.

Once the first months of school, house maintenance and navigating single motherhood were behind me, there were more stirrings in my chest – and in other body parts. It had been so long since I had been touched or held or had Sex. Horniness was knocking at the back door and demanding to come in. In the last few years, David had never seen affection between me and the prince. When he encountered my first after-marriage boyfriend it amazed him that we kissed and laughed and hugged. They were the first displays of love he had seen in his six years of life.

Dating after divorce is more complicated than it used to be. For one thing, there's AIDS and that's scary. I discussed my fears with my doctor and all but fell on the floor when he advised me not to have anal sex. I had never had anal sex. I had no intention of having anal sex. Ever. With anybody. It was going to be a challenge, launching into this brave new world.

It wasn't my habit to immediately jump into bed and it wasn't ever going to be, so sex wasn't my priority concern. What I wanted to understand was how come I was in my mid-thirties but felt like a fourteen year old girl.

I had always had a deep kinship with Hayley Mills. She was a former Disney child actress ("Pollyanna," "The Parent Trap"). She was cute and blonde and snub-nosed but best of all she had this bubbly personality and an irresistible English accent. As Hayley grew older she appeared in movies as a romantic young girl poised for young womanhood. In other words, she played 14 year olds.

When I was 12 I saw a delicious Hayley Mills movie called "The Moon Spinners." It had mystery and suspense and the sea and took place on an island in Greece. You couldn't get much better than that. Except that she was fourteen and had a crush on a dashing mysterious older young man named Mark. Ever heard the name "Mark" in a British accent? MAAAHK. Too marvelous for words. Plus he had a Beatle haircut. I was beyond gone.

At first there's suspense but no romance. But when Mark gets injured Hayley Mills hides him in an old church and --- oh my heart! – Mark kisses her.....gently.....on her *forehead.* Sooo much more romantic than a regular movie star smooch. I sat through two more showings of the "The Moon spinners" just to see that kiss.

THE MYSTERY THAT BINDS ME STILL

I slid backwards when I became single, right back to being giggly and silly and fourteen. Hello again, Hayley Mills.

It embarrassed me to have plunged to such depths but friends were supportive, patient and understanding. Once again, I had to turn to a Competent Friend for help, my friend Mary. She'd already been divorced and into the singles thing for over a year, so it was under her tutelage that I learned the ropes.

Mary went to singles dances, so I went along too. Singles dances are odd anthropological events that produce a myriad of diverse behaviors, dancing being only one of them. Participants viewed these rituals from numerous perspectives. Mary felt perfectly okay about being out there, ready to dance, and if she met someone, fine. She had it all over me in one respect. The first part of the meeting/dancing ritual was to ask each other the nature of our occupations. Mary was a kindergarten teacher and boy was she *in.* Men who met Mary felt comfortable, nostalgic and unthreatened. They reacted to the announcement of her job with warmth. This was not the case for a high school English teacher. Mary brought them sweetness; I seemed to be their worst nightmare.

I felt greatly out of place. I was overwhelmed by all these strangers and the pressure to dance and chat and get to know one another when in most cases I would rather have died first. I also had plenty of opportunity to feel rejected because I wasn't very often asked to dance. One gentleman informed me that this was all my fault.

My difficulties began when my first dance partner inquired what I did and where I worked. Like a fool, I told him. "I'm a high school English teacher," I chirped. I did **not** get a positive response. Most of the gentlemen I danced with answered with one or more of the following:

"Eeuww. It's a dirty job but I guess somebody's got to do it."

"Uh-oh, I'd better watch my grammar."

"I flunked English. I hated it."

"All of my English teachers were creeps."

And so on. These did not sweep me off my feet. Then it occurred to me – these people don't know me; I'm under no obligation to them to tell the truth. So I began trying on a variety of lies:

"I run a series of parachute drops."

"My friend and I own a worm farm."

"I cut holes in blue jeans and sell them in New York boutiques."

And then, the one I was fondest of:

"I'm sorry, but they don't allow me to talk about it."

The other problem was my enthusiastic, creative approach to dancing. When I came to a dance, I was by golly going to dance, with a partner or not. Apparently my dance style was not sedate enough for gentlemen to feel they could approach. One gentleman told me this directly: "If you'll just calm down a bit, more men would dance with you," he said.

THE MYSTERY THAT BINDS ME STILL

I went into my full-blown arrogance. For me, dancing is sacred and holy and free and mine was done with a vigorous spirit. I did NOT turn to him and say "Oh yeah? Well fuck you." I was arrogant, but I was a lady. I simply informed him that I dance the way I dance and if no one had the guts or desire to dance with me, too bad for them.

Together Mary and I presented an enigma for these folks. We came to the dances not to be wares in a meat market, but to enjoy the music and dance. One time we did something that apparently just wasn't *done.* Mary was about to dance with a gentleman but the music that came up was "Do You Love Me?" That was "our" song. I jumped in and asked Mary to dance. Gleefully we did so. This was sacrilege to the men quickly spreading in other directions, shaking their heads.

I admit I was a little jealous of Mary, who had great hair and a gentle demeanor and who was not only an acceptable kindergarten teacher, but quite pretty too. She looked great in pink, and generally ended up finding a relationship or too. I felt like funny sidekick Rhoda to her classy Mary Tyler Moore. Of course this was not the case but I didn't know it at the time. Later when Mary and I talked we discovered she and some of her friends we'd go dancing with sometimes felt jealous of *me.*

Our greatest triumph occurred at a singles dance in Maryland. Mary had to do a bit of dragging me to get there – I'd gotten to the point where I vacillated between finding these dances mildly amusing to moderate torture.

However, I agreed to keep Mary company, and sedately at that. We sat quietly at a table. In no way was I telegraphing invitations for any kind of ranny-gazoo. Still, along came a drunken individual who chose to sit down beside me and whispered in my ear: "I'd ask you to dance, honey," he said, "but my ass hurts."

I had no signs on my back or marks upon my brow, but somehow Mary never got these kinds of guys. Only I did.

To fortify myself for whatever was to come, I got in touch with the Mack Singer within, and I was ready to roll.

"Hey, what's your name?" he said.

"Angela," I answered.

"Oh, say Angela – can I call you Angie – what do you do for a living?"

"I am a submarine commander," I said.

"Nah, c'mon. What do you really do?"

At that moment, to my eternal amazement, Mary stepped into the fray.

"Yes, it's true," she smiled sweetly. Mary has the face of an angel; knowing her, or looking at her, folks would never believe she could tell a lie. I didn't think she was capable of it myself.

"Because Angela is small," Mary continued, "people assume she wouldn't hold such a position. But she does, and she's highly thought of in all the Baltimore and D.C. Naval ranks."

I think Mary actually pulled it off. It was the beginning of a new bond that formed between us. I had discovered a whole new aspect of my long-known friend. Angelic Mary could think fast on her feet, and when the going gets tough, by golly, Mary could lie. What a gal.

Not long after the Maryland dance I decided to actually try my hand at a date.

Since I hadn't dated many or married any Jewish guys, I thought what the heck I'd start with a Jewish Family Services program. They were trying to bring together local Jewish adults. My first date was a phone call. The gentleman wanted to explore conversational possibilities before we actually met. That was ok with me. We talked a while, and then he said, "I hear you are divorced. Would you mind telling me about your marriage and what went wrong so I too may learn?"

I did not call him back to arrange a date.

The second date came from Reading, PA, two hours away. By the time he got to my house he was highly annoyed at the distance he'd had to drive, and told me so. He got out of the car and snapped "You're driving next time."

"Well, you know," I replied, "*some people* prefer to say hello."

I invited him in, and his eyes swept critically over my house. "What you need are some cats," he announced.

I bit my tongue and did not say "What you need is to get out of my house." Suffice to say, a good time was had by none.

Number three was a man twenty years older that I met for dinner. He was a nice guy, dignified and well dressed. He was also a lawyer whose job was to make sure that people scheduled to be evicted from their homes get kicked out. Though it wasn't mine to judge, the thought of his occupation made my stomach curdle. At the end of dinner he was ready to go home; I was ready to go to boogie at an Al-Anon dance. It wasn't a match.

With each new experience I began to leave the Hayley Mills mode and connect with my inner pissed off older broad.

I stopped going to singles dances but went to others not so obviously a market for dreams, lust and meat. Once I was slow-dancing with a gentleman who paused mid-dance. "Um, do you realize you're leading?" he said.

"Yeah I know," I answered him. "You got a problem with that?"

I'd decided that if I was going to be flung among the jetsam of dating, I wasn't going to be the shrinking violet of the past. I got up the gumption one David-less weekend to wander off to a dance club by myself. After dancing to Motown I rested at a table not far from the band. One of the singers looked straight at me while he was singing a love song. I started to do my usual thing, which is to turn around and see what woman he was talking to. I caught myself just in time. I instructed myself to look the man straight in the eye and claim my flirtatious moment. It was corny, but he asked for my phone number and we did go out on a date. The date itself was a disappointment, but hey, I had had my golden moment. I had arrived. I was a strong woman, alone, independent, going to dance clubs and re-writing my own life.

THE MYSTERY THAT BINDS ME STILL

I was also discovering the games that were played in teenage dating had not changed a bit; we may have been adults, but the maturity displayed by some of my dates was no greater than a kid's. I still got lead on and stood up. I still got the same mixed messages – "C'mere, I want you, go away." I was beginning to sour on the whole enterprise when I had the date that that ended all dates.

It was the night before Christmas Eve. I was at a Narcotics Anonymous dance. A rather slick character approached me and asked for a date. I knew better – I could see he was a game player but I was lonely, he was funny and what the hell .He made a date with me for Christmas Eve and never showed up. But that was only the preliminary to the date that ended all dates.

When the phone rang that night I thought it was my lost date, but to my surprise, it was a guy I had known as an acquaintance for a couple of years. He said "Mickie, I hear you're divorced, I just found out, and I know I should be telling you that's terrible but to tell the truth I have been really interested in you for years but you've been married. Now that you're not I'm so happy, and I can't wait to see you. I want to come over tomorrow and bring you a Christmas present."

The red flags were waving, the "don't go there" sirens were sounding in my head. He was going at the speed of light and that wasn't good.......

"Please, Mickie," he pleaded.

"Oh alright," I said.

My admirer arrived on Christmas Day with a huge present and emptied his heart. "I've always been in love with you," he told me. "I can't wait to be with you. When can we have a date? Tomorrow? You're everything I've ever been looking for."

Whoa boy, whoa. Slow down…luckily I was leaving the next day to visit my folks so he'd have to wait a week for a date, and that would give me time to think about what I might be getting into.

A week later upon my return he called. I waited to hear when he'd propose a date, but just as he surprised me with his first call, he astounded me on this one.

"I can't go out with you, Mickie," he said. "During the week you were gone I met my soul mate, the love of my life, and I have to give up dating you."

Wow. A soul mate in only a week. The man moved fast.

I resisted telling him where he could put his date. I wasn't so much hurt or mad, I was speechless. I thought it the height of rudeness; ludicrous, stupid, false, gutless and insincere.

That's IT, I promised myself. I don't play games. I set aside a year just to enjoy my own company and spend more time with friends. NO MORE DATES.

It turned out to be one of the best things I've could have done. It gave me time to become acquainted with me. I learned things about myself I never knew before. I got stronger and more focused, discovered new stuff I liked to do and had a ball going out with women friends. In many ways I felt fulfilled.

I was lonely a lot of the time, but I also had the happy feeling of being free. I had rushed into being with the prince when I was 22; I had barely any time to be "single" in my life. I was grateful for the time to experience it again, even if a lot of it was a pain in the ass. I got through a lot I couldn't imagine I'd be able to – like being all alone for the weekend when David went to his dad's. But after a while I found things I liked to do. On those weekends I'd get up early on a Saturday, dress nicely and go to Central Market for breakfast. A lot of people I knew tended to show up as the morning went on. It was nice just holding court and passing a part of the day.

Once I knew myself better I stood on firmer feet. I learned what my red flags were and swore allegiance to them. I paid attention to the caution signs and danger signals they represented.

After a while, Mary wanted me to go along with her to another singles dance. Reluctantly I went and met a seemingly nice guy – who wanted to take me out on a date. I explained that I wasn't dating and wouldn't give him my phone number, but I'd be willing to take his. I told him I would consider calling him. I thought about it for a week, decided to take the plunge and gave him a call.

He said great, let's arrange a date.

"Nope," I told him. "I'm not ready yet. But I'll be happy to meet you for an hour or two over coffee in a coffee shop. We can talk and see how it goes."

So we passed our two hours of coffee and conversation in the coffee shop. "Now," he said, "are we gonna go out on a date?"

"No, I don't want to date yet, "I said. " I'm not yanking you around. I want to get to know a man gradually, on mutually comfortable turf. Then if we like each other it's time well spent. If the potential is there, we could start to date. For now I'll give you my phone number. I would like to get together with you again and talk some more, take a little more time. If you're interested in doing that, and not dating just for being on a date, hey, call me."

He never called.

But I was okay with that. I had come to know what I wanted and what I didn't. I had taken a hard look at my former marriage and my part in its demise. I realized there were a lot of things I had to change about myself if I wanted to be healthy or attract a healthy-minded man. I had more therapy, went to 12 Step Groups, daily read the Serenity Prayer, and did what I had to do. I examined which changes I was willing and able to make, and what I would just have to accept.

I had one more lesson to learn about the single life. It doesn't matter if you're in your thirties or forties or fifties or nineties, if you become attracted to someone.....you still can develop a full blown, blushing, consuming crush. You think of him all the time, you daydream about him, you wish you could be with him, you imagine what being with him would be like. It's positively humiliating. It amounts to more evidence that we never *really* grow up.

I learned this through personal experience. To my amazement, I developed a crush. I tried not to, but it took on a life of its own. I still wanted to "not date" and was generally suspicious of men. But, despite my efforts to stifle it, I felt wonderful – transcendent, drunk with passion, besotted with joy and awe and fear. My no-dates heart was thumping again. **I had it bad.**

Little did I know he was scared to death of me and wanted nothing more than to get as far away from me as he could. Except....no matter how much he suppressed it he was attracted to me too. It was no use – the festivities were about to begin.

CHAPTER FOURTEEN: DAN

His name was Dan, and he is my husband now.

My second husband, actually, but I don't think of him that way. There's nothing about Dan that isn't entirely first-rate.

I met him through my friend and dancing partner, Mary. She had no intention of getting us together. In fact, we were dating steadily for two years when Mary confessed she'd thought we would never hit it off at all. Two years had passed before she wondered if *maybe* we might last.....fifteen or so years later, we have.

Having us meet for romantic purposes was not in her plans, because for one thing, Mary could not think of two people who seemed to her further apart. It seemed like that to us, too, until we got things settled (which didn't happen any too quickly). I like to think we were like Spencer Tracy and Kathryn Hepburn, battling provocatively, clearly meant for each other at the end. I don't know what Dan thinks about this. It was all rather hard on him.

In any event, I met Dan when Mary took me along to hear his band. He was a drummer who was currently playing classic rock and oldies, my favorite music. This alone intrigued me. I also happened to have a "thing" for drummers. I thought drums were the niftiest instrument of all.

Dan was not just Mary's friend, he was a miracle. When I met Mary, we'd debate about whether or a woman could just be friends with a man. Mary voted "no" to the whole notion. She didn't trust men much at all. This astounded me. I had had male friends all my life. Men who were married to other people, or who had girlfriends or even to whom I had some level of attraction. I protested that when I was friends with a man I valued keeping it that way. Attraction, even when there, does not have to be acted upon. We make choices. But Mary didn't buy it at all.

Thus imagine my surprise a year later when she told me: "I think I have a male friend. His name is Dan."

Wow, I thought. This must be one special man.

Over the years she would tell me all about him. About how he was a talented drummer and an exceptionally sweet man. How he brought her flowers when she was depressed and never asked anything of her than to be his friend. She would tell me about his girlfriends and bands and keep me up to date on how all such things were going. I was impressed.

When I became separated Mary invited me to hear "Sha-Bop," Dan's current band. She and some other friends of ours had long since been band followers, but I had never been free to do that before. I longed to be out among people again - and *dance*.

"Sha-Bop" proved to be an exceptional band. I had a ball on the dance floor; I let go and for the first time in a long time, happily danced. At intermission Sha-Bop sat at a table along with their girlfriends and wives. Mary and the other regulars came over to say hello, this time with me in tow.

Meeting Dan hit me like a brick. The first thing I thought was, My God, I didn't think a man could have a head that big! The second thing was that he absolutely exuded gentleness, sweetness and respect. And my third thought was, that's exactly the kind of guy I *should* be with, but never am.

I didn't know at the time that I was making quite a different impression on Dan. He thought me a "hussy," and a "temptress," who performed strange dances. Because I chose to dance slow dances by myself, he also thought I was "whacked." The thing was, the prince never danced with me and it just so happened that I'd never danced a slow dance and never had been asked to with anyone else. I was tired of following convention and always returning to my seat when the music slowed down. So I danced with myself.

Dan's current girlfriend was along that night. After meeting her I felt profoundly sorry for him. She sat ramrod stiff, joyless and bored. She reminded me of the prince. Hardly at all the sort of woman I thought would suit Dan. "Poor guy," I commented to Mary. "He really ought to dump her."

Months later I returned with Mary and friends to see Dan's band again. The ironing-board-backed girlfriend was still with him. I regarded him even more strongly than before. He regarded me more too – mostly with horror but, to his regret, a little bit of attraction mixed in.

THE MYSTERY THAT BINDS ME STILL

For the next year we'd bump into each other through Mary and sparks would fly alright but mostly they expired in the air. First of all, he pissed me off. I'd try and talk to him pleasantly but no matter what I said he'd lift one eyebrow and answer "Oh?" Okay, I thought, going into defensive stance, you think I'm weird, *watch this.* I got up on my feet and told a story about farts.

There, take that.

Still, I made sure to keep abreast of his situation with the Dead-But-Just-Didn't-Know-It-Yet girlfriend. Mary, angelic and guileless in this matter, had no idea why this subject interested me so much.

For New Year's Eve, Mary and I had a date with each other. She asked if I would mind if Dan came along – he'd just broken up with his girlfriend, she said, and was lonesome. Mary knew he bothered me because he treated me as if I was nuts. "I don't mind," I said reluctantly. "Bring him along. I'll just ignore him."

And I was doing a darn good job of ignoring him, too – all the way in the car, through a movie, even at a dance club, up until Mary asked me to have pity and dance with him. Mary swears to this day that she did no such thing but she's not writing this book, so I'll tell it my way.

It didn't go very well. I'm minute and he is massive; over six feet tall, bearded and broadly built. My arms could not reach around his waist. They kept sliding off. He laughed and said "You ought to dance standing on a chair."

Yeah, well *watch this*, I thought. I pulled a chair onto the dance floor, stood on it and held out my arms. I fully expected him to walk away. To my amazement, he put his arms around me and we danced – with me on that chair – for a good half an hour. When I finally put my feet back on earth, I was mush.

This is a man with guts, with balls, I thought. This is a guy with a sense of humor and adventure. Here's somebody who doesn't step away from the unusual.

I want him.

I wish I could say he called me the next day, but he didn't. I had to pursue him. He was so scared of me I had to have an excuse to do it. Months later I had my chance; when I learned a band needed a drummer, I invited him with me to audition. He said he thought it would work out but he'd check his schedule. "Then," he said, "I'll call Mary."

I refused to be invisible anymore. The shrinking violet was gone. "Well," I replied. "That's just fine, *but Mary is not the one who's inviting you.*"

Thus he was forced to deal with me, and also thus came about our first date.

It was on our second date that the shit hit the fan. I had friends with a house full of jukeboxes I thought he'd like to hear. All went well until we went out to eat. Barely had we placed our orders when Dan looked at me across the table and said "So what do you want, Mickie? Just what is it you're looking for?"

THE MYSTERY THAT BINDS ME STILL

Uh-oh, I thought, I'm with another nut. Where does he come from? The Up- Against-The-Wall School of Dating? But there was something about him - I think his honesty - that prompted me to answer him. I did my best to tell him what I looked for in a relationship. When I asked him the same he delineated a few things and then pronounced "BUT NO WOMAN IS EVER GOING TO COME BEFORE MY MUSIC."

Whoa, I heard that, I thought. Run to the nearest exit. But then he put his arms around me when he walked me to his car. I was mush again. Whatever the future, I knew I wanted to get to know him. In two weeks I'd be having Seder, the special dinner that commemorates Passover. I only invite people who are special to me, and I figured Dan was special. I wanted him to come. One problem presented itself before I invited him, however; I didn't know if he knew I was Jewish, and I figured before I invited him to Seder, that information ought to come first.

We were driving back to my house when I asked him if he knew I was a Jew. "**NO**!" he cried. His hands left the steering wheel and hit the roof.

Nonetheless he promised he'd come Seder. When we pulled into my driveway, *watch this* reared its head. I was mad at him for putting me on the spot back at the restaurant. "So," I said, "are you going to kiss me or what?"

This time he moaned and his head hit the steering wheel. "Just not tonight, ok?" he said. "See ya."

Then he pulled out of the driveway so fast my hair flew up.

I'd scared him again. I didn't know then that I reminded him a great deal of his second wife. She had also been exuberant, playful and an enthusiastic dancer, but ragingly alcoholic. Still, something about me drew him to me just as something about him drew me to him. Despite it all he called me again. I apologized to him for being so forward. He apologized to me for hitting the roof when I told him I was a Jew. He explained that some of his family wasn't particularly partial toward Jewish people and dating me might not go down very well with them.

This excited me – not because of their dislike of Jews - but because of its implication. Apparently he was thinking of dating me and the possible future.

Dan Withers – actually Robert Daniel Withers he is – (except when I can't find him in Wal-Mart, then I have him paged as "Bobby Dan") is the most extraordinary human being I have met in my life. He is not a saint, but he sits to the right of the angels. He has an aura about him that says "Come to me, I like you." Over the years I have seen it repeatedly – strangers come up to him and talk to him, children who don't know him climb in his lap, my friends and family fell in love with him on sight.

Dan came with me to Cincinnati to meet the family when Mom and Dad were in a nursing home. We got there near to the time the home was closing up for the night, so only had a twenty minute visit. When Dad – who had always been courteous but distant with my boyfriends, met Dan, he hugged him immediately and said "You're a hunk to get hold of!" I never saw my father behave like that before – there was just something about Dan.

When my mother walked us out to say goodbye she announced right in front of Dan: "You know that when your father dies, I intend to kill myself." I had warned him about Mom but a warning doesn't compare to getting a full blast of her head-on. He stood his ground, though. The blessed man didn't blink an eye. He treated her with utter respect and courtesy and she fell entirely in love.

I've heard Dan described as a big teddy bear. It's a pretty good portrait, but it doesn't begin to truly depict this remarkable man. Physically he resembles Paul Bunyan, the legendary frontier giant. Some find him intimidating, which he can pull off well when he wants to; he has a deep voice and when he is angry his tone is sharp and his eyes flash. But for the most part the teddy bear is what comes through.

I am also fond of his sexy lips and caramel-brown eyes.

Dan is an endless joy – funny, whimsical and outrageous to a degree that often rivals me. He is extremely playful and we play a great deal of the time. We often wrestle, play tag in parking lots and egg each other on. I love his strange and unpredictable mind which produces considerable nonsense. Not only is he a lover of life and the human race, he is one of the few people I have ever known to truly treat others as he would wish to be treated himself.

Dan has taught me a great deal about patience, trust and respect. I admire him tremendously; he fairly drips testosterone and would easily be described as "a man's man" yet he loves flowers and has been known to sleep occasionally with a favorite stuffed bear. And if anyone has a problem with that, he truly doesn't care. He is immensely independent and walks his own path, yet is gentle and unfailingly considerate.

My father would say Dan was a "good egg" – which was Dad's highest praise. Then he'd probably add: "He's got a heart as big as he is." I admire Dan because he has survived some very rough times. Earlier in his life, he tells me, he was a very different person. Mary has talked about him in the days of her early acquaintance – she says he was so angry it scared her to sit next to him. According to Dan he was rough and crude and sometimes mean. You couldn't swear it by me. I don't doubt he is telling the truth. But by the time I came along he was deep into Dan phase two.

When he came to the realization that his rough attitude wasn't what he wanted, he did something about it. Rather than reach for a bottle or a gun or just keep on as he had been, he went to professionals for help, even though some of his friends and family regarded them as professional as witch doctors. Dan broke the mold. He worked to change in any way that he could.

THE MYSTERY THAT BINDS ME STILL

I also admire him because he is a dedicated, devoted Christian. He doesn't just talk the talk, he walks the walk. Even though Christianity is not my path, I think it's a good one and not an easy one to follow. I have seen Dan grow in his spirituality and his church community. I sometimes accompany him to church, which is filled with good folks. Dan and I respect each other's paths, but sometimes we get to talking about our differences, and the air can get pretty hot.

Overall, Dan is a simple man. He enjoys simple pleasures – sitting in a comfortable rocking chair, eating a good apple pie, adventuring about the countryside. His values are simple as well. Whoever that Greek guy was (I forget his name) who wandered around trying to find an honest man, he could have stopped if he had met Dan.

He is a gift to everyone he meets.

Contrary to the prince, Dan truly accepts who I am. He's been with me through some whoppers - some sick, some scary, and some fun. He likes to listen to my stories and knows them by heart. He accepts that my sleep is always extreme; from none at all to marathon hours at a time. If I wander off in the wrong direction when the car is clearly parked somewhere else (that's A.D.D. in action), he just laughs and guides me back to where I should be. He could care less about how I hang washrags, or how long I'm on the phone, or if I want to go out with a friend. He allows me to make mistakes, gives me space and wants only for me to be content.

It's taken me a while to trust who he, and our relationship, is. At the first sign of his occasional grumpiness my danger signals come up. Is this it? Is this when it begins?- runs through my head. Then I talk myself into reviewing reality. Yes, Dan is human. Yes, he makes mistakes. And no, every marriage I'm involved in is not fated to go sour after six or seven years. Whew. Check.

I've had plenty opportunity to see Dan's humor and acceptance in action. One winter night (under the influence of some strong A.D.D. impulsivity), I drove right up onto a cement island in the middle of the street. I waited for Dan to issue the verbal punishment I deserved. Panicking, I shouted "What do I do now?" all the while cringing in my seat.

"Just get back down the same way you got up," he answered mildly. "Don't worry about it, dear; it was just a cheap thrill."

Early on, Dan observed some episodes where my judgment was clouded or when I lost control. It didn't startle him one night when I crawled under a table in a dance club and slept on the floor while the band was playing. I was tired at the time and also manic so I thought lying underneath a table to sleep made sense. Months later, I asked him how he could be with me when I'm unstable. Also, how could he continue to be with me, knowing there would surely be times I'd be unstable again? His answer was as simple as he is: "Faith," he said.

One of the things I particularly enjoy about Dan is that he is not easily fazed. This leaves me plenty of room to be eccentric. Also, Dan eggs me on. He challenges me to do things like paint my car, which I did with little paintings and designs, poetry and sayings. When we were first dating I showed him what I'd been working on that day, which was a big mural of a tree covering my entire front door. He just stood there looking at it and said: "I will never be surprised at anything you do again."

He's been as good as his word.

I am not easily fazed either, and so we are perpetually launched into a battle of who can faze who. Sometimes, however, he worries. He's seen me in some mild to not-so-moderate doozies so he fears I'll completely "lose it" someday. One night he was snoring terribly. Nothing I did could persuade him to stop. Okay, I thought to myself, fair is fair. If you're going to snore, I'm going to sing. As soon as I started singing, Dan woke up, alarmed. "No dear, don't, he pleaded. "Don't sing. Don't do it!"

He thought I had lost it for good.

We spent years and a lot of gas traveling back and forth between our homes, 45 miles away. Lord knows I had my hesitations about marriage, coming from my horror of an experience. Dan had been married, twice, both times to alcoholic wives. We had been in Al-Anon "recovery" but agreed we needed some intensive work regarding ourselves. For two years we were in couple's therapy, banging around our old baggage and sending it on its way.

Our love didn't "blossom" immediately because we took our time to get to know each other as friends. That was Dan's idea, not mine. But he stood steadfast. Two months passed before he would kiss me. A week after that I told him "I think I probably love you."

"I think I probably love you, too," he said.

It was going on six years until Dan felt truly comfortable enough to commit to marriage. He was well worth the patience and the wait. The proposal, however, didn't go the way he'd planned.

It was near Christmas and David was doing a special favor, babysitting at a Narcotics Anonymous meeting. Dan and I went to lunch, returning to walk very quietly down the hallway and wait silently outside the door. We wanted to hear how David handled the babysitting. We got a big kick out of hearing David competently instruct the children that they could keep one toy out but they had to put all the other toys away.

Then one of the mothers came to get her child and we stepped aside. David still didn't know we were there. He was bursting with secret news to share with this stranger. He would never in a million years have given it away, but he didn't know we were there. "Guess what?" he said to the woman. "My mother's boy friend is going to ask her to marry him!"

There weren't any cats left in the bag so when we got home, Dan was obliged to do the deed. Down he went on his knees, offered a diamond ring, and asked me to marry him.

THE MYSTERY THAT BINDS ME STILL

It was a long way from "I'm tired of hearing you bitch. Set the date."

Our wedding was a little irregular, too. We saw no reason to do anything elaborate or spend money we didn't have. Our invitations asked guests to bring a lawn chair and some potluck to share and we'd provide non-alcoholic drinks. It was easy-going and fun and personally meaningful for us both. Dan had a minister to stand up for him and I had my cousin Leah who wrote a beautiful Jewish ceremony. We had a friend to play "Sheebeg Shemore" (an Irish tune about fairies) for our wedding march. We had another friend sing and play "Oh Danny Boy", the favorite song of both my father and Dan's. We invited my father and mother, and Dan's father, all of whom had passed away, to be among us that day.

I wore a genuine Victorian nightgown and a wide-brimmed high flowered hat; Dan was in a grey suit and a matching flea-market find, a grey high-top hat upon his head. The owners' dogs ran around us and nearly knocked over the wine. My brother Barry was wearing the Harley-Davidson t-shirt I'd bought him. Some of my students were there. It meant a great deal to me to hear people say it was the only wedding they had truly enjoyed. It was an all-around love-feast, just perfect for the way we wanted to begin.

Except of course, things went wrong. There was no problem with our accommodations – we were right where we wanted to be. Years ago I had discovered Spoutwood Farm, a beautiful placed owned by my friends Lucy and Rob. I came anytime, even when they weren't there, (with their permission) just to soak it in. It was very serene. The day I learned I was divorced Spoutwood was where I came to be alone with the news. I noticed a large meadow with two old willow trees standing opposite and apart – with boughs meeting, tenderly bent toward each other, in the middle.

Hah, I thought. What a perfect place to get married.

And so it was all arranged with Lucy and Rob, if I was ever to marry again the ceremony would be there. In fact I told Dan that and took him to see it on our third date. Dan being Dan, he took it in stride.

A week before the wedding, the old willow tree on the left crashed and died. The night before the wedding, all three of us stayed in their bed and breakfast, Dogwood House. It was old and charming and incredibly hot. I couldn't drop off at all. Dan claimed he wasn't nervous but screamed loudly several times in his sleep. We were in a century-old bed, built for smaller people – Dan's feet and half his calves were hanging out from the bottom of it. We woke up in the morning to a day that was 99 degrees in temperature and 98 percent humidity. It was ungodly. None of this bothered us a bit.

We spent our honeymoon night at home. It wasn't sexy, but the bed fit and it was air conditioned.

I have a fantasy that Dan ought to be brought into schools, like they do with characters such as Scotty the Firedog and the Safety Police. Dan wouldn't teach about fire or safety. Instead, he would be a living representation of what a truly good human being can be. To some degree my dream came true. For a time Dan was head custodian at an elementary school, universally loved by all the children – teachers and staff too.

Perhaps I am proudest of him for rising above the closed thinking of his earlier life. Although he found it difficult – although he struggled with the decision for several days – he agreed to be the King of the Fairies for the 2001 Fairy Festival at Spoutwood Farm. That was Big stuff for a man that was raised in Mennonite/Brethern Ephrata. I, of course, was the Queen.

Once I asked my parents what kept them together and in love all those 53 years. Their answer -"We laugh together a lot."

We do too. I don't know if we'll get 53 years to do it, but if that's the formula for lasting marriage, we'll live happily ever after.

Amen.

CHAPTER FIFTEEN: I BECOME AN ORPHAN
AND GAIN A GHOST

I don't relate very well to numbers so I don't think of things occurring in particular years. For the life of me I can't think of the year Dan and I were married, although I know the day (July 27th). Sometimes I can remember years that had big round numbers, like my last ten years teaching public school went from 1990 to 2000. And of course I remember David was born in 1983, 2:20 in the morning on September 17th. I further recall that it was Yom Kippur, and my Ob/Gyn was an Orthodox Jew who insisted on hooking me up to pitosin while I labored away and he left and went to services.

So I don't know the days or years my parents died, and I don't care to. I know Dad's been gone close to eleven years, and Mom about two years after that. Such as it goes, that's the math.

Someone once said "the world's a strange place without your parents in it" and whoever he/she was, they were right. I still claim the right to be somebody's baby. But with my parents gone, I'm nobody's baby anymore. It leaves a hole. The love of spouses and children are important, but it's a different thing. Parental love offers shining admiration. You can bathe in the center of their universe, be the light of their lives. They get the double prints of every dumb picture you take. Who else will want them, or look at them with such delight?

THE MYSTERY THAT BINDS ME STILL

Dad's dying took close to three years, which it should not have. According to My Brother the Doctor, it should have happened a lot earlier than that. Mom broke the news that Dad had congestive heart disease – that was in late winter of whatever year. I told her I'd be there the coming summer. But when I talked to Jon he told me I ought not to wait that long. As it happened I came early spring at Passover.

For several days we all sat around and never mentioned that Dad was sick. It was odd but not untoward in my family where emotions were generally suppressed (unless you were Mom and then you were allowed to have a whole mess of 'em). On my last day there I could stand it no more, and motioned Dad into a bedroom.

I tried my best not to cry. The only way I could think to bring it up was to say, "Daddy, I don't know when I'll see you again."

Dad looked at me clearly and spoke some reassuring but rather startling words. "I know what I've got," he said. "I'm not afraid to die. But I can promise you I am not going until I'm ready."

Dad was nothing if not a stubborn cuss and I believed him. Still, it took me aback to hear him declare himself in control of his own death. But that's how he was. His favorite poem, "Invictus," reflected his philosophy and he quoted it often: "I am the master of my fate, I am the captain of my soul."

Thus he declared promise number one.

Despite my efforts, I began to choke up. "Daddy, I'll miss you, "I said.

"You won't have to," he flung back at me without hesitation and entirely sincere. "I'll be right here. I'll always be right here."

That was promise number two and it spooked me out. I knew that Dad always kept his promises and always said what he meant. But neither of my parents were very mystical. Mom was not so at all – only rational, logical proof made sense to her. Dad was a little more off the beam, enjoying his fairies and such. But like Mom, the religion he practiced was practicality. Both of my folks had grown up in the era of assimilation, free thinking and turning from traditional, "superstitious" ways. They took pride in being practical, and demanded that our lives be designed from it. Thus we denied heaven; forbidden to eat no more than one chocolate from the candy box a day.

I had never heard either of them profess belief in life after death. "You live on in the memories of you friends and your children," Mom would say. Dad on the other hand tended to believe in the Divine- I remember him saying that he had proof of God whenever he gazed at a tree – but Mom was an atheist, through and through. I never heard Dad pray except at the Passover Seder. As the lead male, it was his job to lead us through the Haggadah, the Passover prayer book. He got pretty impatient with the whole process. One year he skipped an entire chapter, announcing "The rest of this is mere conjecture." Thus he cut the Seder time in half. Between the two of them, spirituality was not a priority.

THE MYSTERY THAT BINDS ME STILL

On this day, however, Dad was speaking about a highly mystical matter, and did so in his-almost angry, no nonsense, and direct way. "I'll be here," he had said. "I'll always be here." We left it at that.

Dad made good on his first promise. Gradually he grew sicker and more uncomfortable. Our phone conversations centered on whether or not he'd breathed well that day. He kept himself going as long as he could, but he was having problems coping and Mom was having problems coping even more. She had to deal with her own slowly draining grief as well as be a nurse on constant alert. It ended up taking a toll on her, too.

It was a relief when the Dad we knew still surfaced. He used his humor even in the saddest times – like when he couldn't eat. Mom would cook his favorite things. All he could manage was a few bites; he always left quite a bit of food on his plate. Mom would beg him to finish. But he couldn't. "This isn't for me anymore," he'd tell her.

"I'm saving it up to feed the wee folk."

Considering Mom's exhaustion and Dad's condition, they agreed to go to a nursing home. They took up residence in a tiny room with two beds. Mom's one pleasure was a little refrigerator where she could keep her beloved Cokes. Other than that, she was miserable. The only place that would accept them was the Orthodox Jewish home. She hated their religiously-oriented rules. What really got to her was the day the resident rabbi raided their room. Outraged, he searched the little refrigerator and removed her stash of ham.

We had never "kept kosher" so at home we ate ham and bacon without a thought. But Mom would never, never serve pork. One day she told me why. It wasn't because of religious conviction. It was because she had once shared a hospital room with a girl who had trichinosis and Mom never forgot the horror of it. This led to an amusing episode during a meet-the-in-laws occasion when Jon was engaged to be married.

Ruth came from a Catholic family. Her mother, a very nice lady, had gone out of her way to lay on a spread. She served all kinds of good things, including a platter with three different kinds of meat. I took some chicken and roast beef and a small slice of a pale meat I couldn't identify. I took a bite and was surprised. "What is this meat?" I asked. "I don't think I've ever tasted it before."

"It's pork," Ruth's mother said pleasantly. Then it hit her. Her hand flew to her mouth. "Oh my God!!" she said.

We all assured her not to worry, there had been no offense.

Dad wasn't always lucid while in the nursing home. All kinds of things were happening to him, his body and his brain. After three years he became gradually incontinent, wheelchair bound, deaf and couldn't breathe without oxygen. But he wasn't in any mood to die and he hung on. He was keeping Promise Number One.

But in early January of whatever year, he turned to Mom, and declared he was "ready."

THE MYSTERY THAT BINDS ME STILL

"Don't let them give me any medication or food," he instructed her. When the food tray came in Dad said it smelled so good but he had to be strong. Eventually he fell into a coma. Three days later he died.

He had kept Promise Number One.

I flew to Cincinnati, but I don't remember very much of what happened. There was no funeral; Dad had given his body to science. The hospital would cremate him along with other bodies – there would be no ashes, and neither Mom nor Dad wanted a memorial service. For me, that was difficult; I needed a sense of closure.

Now Mom was alone – and alive. Despite her threats she didn't commit suicide – which was ironic, because Dad just had.

When I returned home, my rabbi conducted a memorial service in my living room, where I was surrounded by friends. It helped. Most of my grief had been expressed during the years of his dying. By that time I was largely numb. I was in awe of how Dad had kept Promise Number One. I didn't give a thought to the Promise Number Two, nor expect any events yet to come.

Several days after I returned home I noticed that the desk chair in my office kept gravitating, unseen, to the middle of the room. I thought nothing of it; I figured David was doing it for some reason of his own.

Then objects showed up in different places than where I'd put them, or they disappeared. I asked David if he was doing this. He said not.

That was The Beginning. For the next several years, it was like my house was under siege. I never knew what would happen next. We'd leave the house with the thermostat at a normal temperature; we'd return home and it was turned down to sixty or up to 90 degrees. Faucets turned on and off by themselves. Soap bottles, unbidden, would go pop. Doors slammed. Alarms went off when they weren't set. My radio played by itself. David didn't know about it and I didn't tell him. The majority of this stuff occurred when he was asleep or out of the house.

I shared these experiences with no one but Dan. I assumed most people would think I was nuts. Sure enough, a friend asked me how I could tell these manifestations weren't part of my disease.

Because such manifestations don't occur in any of my disorders, that's why, and there's no indication of any other disorder present. As a bi-polar two I don't, and never have had, psychotic features. Throwing up, and the general meebie-jeebies, yes. Hallucinations or delusions, no.

I didn't wander the house whispering "Dad, is that you?" but I suspected strongly that it was. He always kept his promises. I didn't know if he intended for the poltergeist act to reassure or amuse me, but I found it unsettling instead. These things just weren't supposed to happen, but they were happening. Knowing that, it left me feeling crazy – again.

One night at 3 a.m. a music box I hadn't wound in years started to play all by itself. I turned on a light. It was still going around and around. It was playing "Amazing Grace." Perhaps the intent had been to comfort me, but I was scared to death. I stayed up the rest of the night, barely breathing, waiting for What Might Come Next. I wanted to call someone, but whom? Ghostbusters? They were nothing but a movie back then.

David still wasn't noticing anything untoward and I wasn't about to tell him. Everything appeared to get my particular attention. After the music box incident, I was so shaken that I told what I was experiencing to a few folks I could trust. To my amazement, they told me stories of their own experiences in return. Several of them talked about seeing their parents after they had passed on. One friend did not agree. She said "People often believe they see their loved ones after they die."

But I found myself wondering, if so many people report seeing dead loved ones, might it be *because they see them?* I tried to believe I had underground caverns or subterranean currents and I suppose swamp gas would have come next. Unfortunately the rational explanations did not make sense.

The house was so active it could have been alive. Nothing stayed anymore on my walls. Paintings, prints, wooden thingamajigs, stained glass, photographs, you name it, they all suddenly took to removing themselves from the walls. I know I certainly didn't do it, and David didn't either. As in the other activities, most of it occurred when he was spending the weekend with his father or slumbering somewhere else.

The object-on-the-wall removals were done with class. I rarely saw them move, but overnight or when I was alone in the house after I went out, something would have fallen to the floor. Nothing ever broke, glass or not. Nails and wall hangers were always left neatly in the walls. They never accompanied the objects, they were never bent in any way or misshapen, missing, loose or gone. The only logical, scientific answer to the way they fell was that someone was lifting them off their hangers and gently depositing them on the floor. Except, there wasn't anything corporeal doing it.

By that time I was distressed. Like Dorothy and her companions in the woods, I did believe in spooks, I did believe in spooks. I could come to no other conclusion.

My brother Barry is an Unbeliever of Great Renown. In fact, he helped edit and write a book of essays debunking the paranormal. He lives in China now where everyone believes in ghosts but he has yet to have been converted. He spent a year teaching at a university in Virginia, close enough that he could visit us often. The first weekend he visited things were falling off the walls all over the place. Dad was trying to get his attention, I'm sure, but I was loath to mention this to Barry. I doubt it would have gone over very well.

It all came to a head when the cleaning woman came to the house. She was the mother of one of David's classmates, she did great work and she was cheap. David and I went shopping for a bit and left her to do her thing. We were only gone a short time but upon return her car was no longer in the driveway.

Coming through the garage the first thing I saw was a note on the kitchen counter. It was signed by our cleaning lady and said "Call me right away." So I did.

Her voice was shaking; she sounded as if she was ready to cry. "I don't know what to tell you, I hardly know how to do it. All I can tell you is what happened."

She had been cleaning in the bathroom, she reported, when she heard a crash from the dining room. She dashed over and saw that a photograph there had come off the wall – yet none of the glass was broken, the metal frame wasn't bent and the wall hanger was still untouched in the wall. As she was examining the photo, she heard another crash coming from the living room. A gargoyle on a pedestal had fallen to the floor. While she was looking at that, she heard a *pop* behind her and the removable top from the bird cage flew straight up in the air. She dropped everything, she said, and "got out of there."

It would be just like Dad to be playful with an unsuspecting person. All I could do was apologize and told her that such events were not unusual in my house.

In realized it was time to tell David, before the cleaning lady's son spread it all over school. We had one of The Hardest Talks I ever had to give. Not about sex, but about ghosts. "David, sit down," I said, putting my arm around him. "I have to tell you we are not alone in this house.

He was plenty surprised and a little bit scared, but he took the news pretty well.

The next day when he came home from school he thanked me for telling him when I did. The kids were talking about it all day, he said. The topper was a boy who approached him at lunchtime. "**DAMN,** David," he'd exclaimed. "Your house is *HAUNTED*!"

The "haunting" went on nearly three years until my nerves couldn't take it anymore. But I was clueless about what to do. I wasn't Catholic so that eliminated an exorcism. Someone gave me the phone number of a psychic. She declined to help me other than offering to read me a spell over the telephone. "I wish people would stop calling me about these things," she said. "I'm tired of banishing some poor murdered soul."

Another woman told me to burn lots of sage. It was a cleansing tool, she said.

I figured I had nothing to lose, so I bought a couple bouquets of dried sage and let them smolder while I walked around the house. I felt extremely foolish. I was also horrified to find that burning sage smells just like marijuana, and the odor of it lingered everywhere. The prince brought David home just as I was cleaning up. "Hmmmm," he sniffed. "Back to the sixties, are we?"

Nonetheless, I was resolved to seek peace. Dan suggested I contact his cousin, who was a fulltime practicing psychic. He didn't do this type of work, he told me, but he knew someone who did.

THE MYSTERY THAT BINDS ME STILL

She was a reiki master who lived out of town. I didn't know anything about reiki and didn't want to. I was just desperate to reclaim my house.

Thus I came to be involved in the strangest adventure of my life.

The psychic was a very nice lady. She brought in holy water, sage and a few other herbs. First, she said, I was to sit quietly while she ran her hands all over my body, healing me with prayers and holy water. Then she went from room to room, throwing holy water and saying prayers and receiving, she said, impressions in her mind.

"It's your father," she told me. "He's come to tell you that he was wrong, that there is a spirit life, and he wants you to know that. The last thing I saw was a white-haired, smiling dragon, which smiled at you and flew away. Now he, and your house, will be at peace."

A white-haired smiling dragon; yep - it sure sounded like Dad to me!

The house felt different when the reiki master left. The tension was gone. I immediately relaxed. There were no more incidents - until Dan and I got ready to be married.

I elected not to have a maid or matron of honor. I asked David to stand up with me instead. Several nights before the wedding, I was ironing on letters to make David a t-shirt saying "BEST SON." When done, I put the iron back in the bathroom. We lived in a ranch house where the distance of the living room from the bathroom was maybe three seconds. I had just been admiring the lettering; they were a deep crimson, so bright they seemed to glow. When I returned from the bathroom, the letters weren't visible anymore. The t-shirt had been turned upside down.

Hours later when I turned on the bedroom lights in my bedroom, it became apparent something was wrong. Only a dim blue light from Dan's lamp came on. My lamp was the one connected to the light switch; but not this night. The lamps had been switched to different nightstands.

Dan and I figured it was Dad letting us know he knew we were getting married and came to say hello. Everything that happened that evening was specifically aimed at David, Dan and me. I believe Dad was telling us he approved of our new family.

There were a few more curious incidents throughout the years. Once, the hands on a clock completely disappeared. Another time Dan's heavy antique mirror showed up in the office, instead of in the basement where it had been stored. We took it all in stride.

Mom was never told any of this. I assumed she wouldn't believe me. But before she died she told me that she had seen Dad, standing right beside her with his hand on her shoulder. "I haven't told this to anybody," she whispered. "But I saw him. He was there."

"You did see him, Mom," I told her. "He *was* there."

She was shaken and unsuited to such thoughts. When I told her about what I experienced, I'm not sure how she took it. But it seemed like it gave her a measure of comfort.

Mom lived for two years following Dad's death. Instead of killing herself, she willed herself to live. She had been on medication to lower her blood pressure; it made her so groggy all she could do was sleep. She chose not to take it anymore, and let whatever circumstances occur. After a while they did. She had a stroke.

For a year afterward, this woman who we siblings had looked upon as "weak" proved she was anything but. She didn't bounce back after the stroke, but she lurched forward, determined to get agile enough to return to her own room. She was in the hospital for several months and she had hours of physical therapy. She worked hard to get back what life she could.

I began to look at Mom with a new perspective. It was a revelation. Between my parents, Dad wasn't really the "strong one." Mom was.

When the second stroke came, it was terminal. While she lingered she was kept on oxygen. It was only to make her more comfortable while she was in a coma. When I returned to Cincinnati, Jon and I joined forces to insist that no other life-promoting procedures be done. Mom was sleeping now, on her way to be with her beloved Mack. We wanted nothing to get in the way.

Mom never promised me she'd watch over me as Dad had, and I've never received a sign that she's there. The night I came back home from

Cincinnati, however, another of my music boxes played all by itself. The song was "Love Story."

I knew it was a message. Mom and Dad are together again.

THE MYSTERY THAT BINDS ME STILL

CHAPTER SIXTEEN: THE PSYCH WARD – AGAIN

Having left teaching, I was flying without a net. I did have a job to go to – something that seemed vaguely like working and being a help with teens – but I really didn't know what I was doing, or if it would last. I took a vast pay cut, less than half of what I was earning before. But I put on a brave smile, mumbling things about a new life and risk taking and how it was all going to turn out alright.

I was scared to death.

In mid-June I reported to a "wrap-around service" for training. If you don't know what a wrap-around service is you have lived a charmed life. If you do know what a wrap-around service is, you have been acquainted with disaster and misery; the kind that can only be associated with the "at-risk" child.

Wrap around programs are designed to have a therapist working with a child both at home and at school. A behavioral specialist may be involved as well as a behavioral support person, otherwise known as a TSS (therapeutic staff support). A TSS works with a plan developed by the child's therapists. The TSS must accompany the child wherever necessary, "monitoring and guiding behavior." These behaviors are usually amazing, astonishing, and downright appalling. TSS training may as well be a hearty "Good Luck."

To be fair, folks who wish to be a TSS do get trained. How effective the training is depends

Mickie R. Singer

on what the prospective TSS is ready to face. I, for one, had no idea that I would have to learn maneuvers meant to physically subdue a raging child. This child, I might add, was to be of any size, and the maneuvers were to be equally sufficient – no matter the TSS' size, which in my case was practically munchkin.

And entirely without a muscle to boot.

I did my best, I really did, but the only reason I passed was by the good graces of my trainer. Upon returning home, I immediately jumped on David and Dan. I used my best subduing maneuvers. David broke out of the first one in two seconds saying "What the hell are you trying to do, Mom?" Dan wouldn't even give me the dignity of breaking out. He just looked at me and walked away.

After also attempting mastery of CPR and other moves, none of which did I get, I was turned loose on the child the agency had picked. The devil had whispered in their ear because I was paired with Bobby, a 14 year old boy so incorrigible that not only had he run through every TSS he'd had in two years, but he had also been completely unsuccessful in all existing programs, from juvenile prison to junior boot camp to reform school. What magic I was supposed to work with him, I had no clue.

Nonetheless, there we were, smiling warily at each other from across the room. Bobby was tall and rangy and easy-going except for when he got riled. Then he went ballistic. He was absolutely convinced he never had to do anything he didn't want to. Later, I asked him how he got through all the punishments rained upon him for his disobedience; at the prison, for instance. "I figured it didn't matter what they did to me," he told me. "I knew eventually they'd send me home."

And he was right. I found it hard to argue with Bobby's logic. In fact I stopped doing it at all. Instead, I introduced him to the logic of my own.

The first day we were together I asked Bobby what he would like to do (smooth move, I thought, establish a friendly relationship with him on his ground.) He said he wanted to go mountain hiking. So we did, tromping off the paths all over the deep, deep woods. I was having a great time. Bobby was very bright and truly knew his mountain lore. He was entertaining me, identifying all the flora and fauna and explaining how they came to be, to boot. I was so involved that it was quite some time – a little past the time it was obvious that we were lost – before I considered the wisdom of letting him drag me into the woods.

Bobby assured me safety was soon to be found. The woods thinned, and we came to a hill filled with cornfields, at the bottom of which was a ditch. There was no other way out than to go down the hill and over the ditch. Bobby, young and agile, just hopped across it. I, however, fell in it and couldn't get out. He could easily have left me there, but our bond of trust began when he pulled me out.

When I got back to the office I told everyone what a happy time I had spent with him.

I was warned. "Just wait," they told me. "He hasn't *tested* you yet."

He did, the very next day.

I reported to his trailer at the appointed time, ten o'clock. His door was open but there was no response to my knock. I found him fast asleep, covered with a blanket on the couch.

I must have nudged and nagged at him for nearly an hour, trying all possible permutations of "Bobby, wake up." He was not paying me any attention. He was not making a move.

Sensitive to my newness as a TSS, as well as Bobby's well known discontent; the agency director had given me his cell phone number. He told me if things got rough to call. Finally I did. I sat there on the opposite couch, waiting for the Marines to come and kick ass. The director burst through the door, and in full military voice, demanded that Bobby get up. Bobby sat up – just barely - but that was as far as he was willing to go. Despite all threats he remained steadfast on the couch. Disgusted, the director gave up and left.

After that impressive display of military-like might I was apparently on my own. There was nothing I could go on but instinct, so I sat on the floor next to the couch, my face just a few inches from Bobby's. "Listen," I said, "if you don't get up off that couch I'm going to pick my nose. Furthermore, I'm going to pick *your* nose."

That boy was off the couch quicker than you can say "Aunt Bea's wax" and soon we were on our way.

THE MYSTERY THAT BINDS ME STILL

I had stumbled onto the best methodology I could use – let him believe I'm crazy. It kept him off balance and made him laugh. It kept him guessing, too. We still had our difficult times, but he was one of the best playmates I'd ever had and that summer was a happy time. We wandered through parking lots, counting the license plates from different states. We talked to each other in different accents. Bobby loved messing around in water. We visited quite a few of streams and lakes. He delighted in scaring me with his collections of water snakes.

I monitored Bobby's behavior all right, but not to very much avail. At fourteen he was already a deeply damaged individual. His only happiness came in taking care of animals and being as wild as he could be. There were lots of reasons why Bobby was the way he was, not the least of which was his mother. She could care less about my – or the agency's – efforts. A TSS was a free babysitter, as far as she was concerned. In her eyes Bobby was worthless and worse and she told him so. Often. In that brief summer Bobby and I were together, I don't know if he came away with anything useful but if nothing else he knew that there was at least one female adult who thought he was great.

During my TSS duties I was also treated to several days work in the juvenile jail. It was a fully locked down, secure facility in which there was allowed absolutely no ranny-gazoo. To my astonishment, before they went anywhere the young inmates lined up military-style, one arm's length away from each other against the wall. My personal favorite was the bathroom formation. Each kid had an assigned rule to loudly call, beginning with "No urinating on the seat, SIR!" to "No masturbating in the stalls, SIR!"

When school began I was assigned a new child whom I would have to accompany from class to class. It bored me, which always gets me depressed. Even more, it horrified me to see the students getting away with unacceptable behavior, while I was in no position to do anything about it. After a while I began to get panic attacks and had to go home. Thus came the end of my career as a TSS.

My next endeavor was substitute teaching. It didn't work too well. I was too fresh from being a "real" teacher to accept that I wasn't a continuing part of a school community, or that in most classes I was a warm body who rarely got to really teach.

In March I got a phone call from the director of a local mental health association, offering me the position of director of education. I thought the angels from Heaven had kissed me on the eyes. I couldn't have a job more perfect for me, combining my interests in both education and mental health. It was, my friend Michael wrote, "Life poetry."

The agency was founded in the 50's to provide education, advocacy and assistance to the mentally ill, the general community and to friends and families. Under my aegis was everything from organizing and/or leading support groups, creating

THE MYSTERY THAT BINDS ME STILL

workshops, programs and presentations, setting up places for screening to be done on mental health day, handling the press and publicity, writing a column for the local paper, going to schools and conferences and anywhere I was asked to help illuminate and eliminate the stigma against mental illness.

I also attended many dinners consisting of dry, unpalatable food, especially what a colleague referred to as "non-profit chicken."

It kept me busy and I loved it, for close to two years. But it also took its toll. I might work 12-15 or more hours in a day. I was often on the other end of the phone listening to anguished siblings and parents. The more programs I created, the more I had to work, and the more I worked, the more I saw that the stigma toward mental illness had no end in sight..

It was quite a different experience from what I was accustomed. In the classroom I more or less called the shots. It was my own little kingdom, which was one of the reasons I fared so well there. There was occasional interference – parents' negative phone calls, the principal picking up trash in the hallway and always stopping in my room to throw it in my wastebasket (he didn't fool anyone; it was an obvious spy tactic. My students and I giggled every time.). There were days I was "observed" and had to attend mind-numbing "in-service days" as well. But for the most part I was my own boss and did what I did in my own way.

But in agency work I was under someone else's rule. It took considerable getting used to.

The work fed my creativity, but I sometimes felt like I was packed inside a box.

After a time my spirit bucked and I had to break free. Still, I had a plan – and brave thoughts. I would take my retirement money and build a consultant business of my own. I spent thousands on publicity and mailings and stamps, bought a computer and prepaid the rent for months ahead. I had finally realized that I couldn't – and never could – function inside of a box. So why did I keep banging my head against one?

I'd always wanted to be Johnny Appleseed. You know, go wandering, planting apples and going to dinner in a lot of friendly people's houses; or something to that effect. I wasn't at ease with other people's choices toward what I was to wear or how I was to behave. It always seemed odd to me that our culture looks down on those who are inventive or outside of the norm. Yet many of those we are taught to admire – Benjamin Franklin, Amelia Earhart, and Albert Einstein – for example, were all people who did not fit in the box. As an English teacher, I was required to teach Shakespeare, Emerson and Thoreau – none of them fit in a box, either. Yet I couldn't act like Ben Franklin, Thoreau or Amelia Earhart. I was to teach, not to model – which I found impossible because I model what I teach.

I don't know what the answer is to this quandary. I guess if you're a genius or disappear or become unknown, not fitting in the box becomes a fitting thing.

THE MYSTERY THAT BINDS ME STILL

I took an enormous gamble on my consultant business. I was convinced that I had hit on what I was supposed to do at last. Then our governor slashed the funds available to human services, and I took a nosedive – my retirement money was gone, I wasn't getting any jobs and I was dead broke.

With each disappointment, I spiraled down a little more. Then I took a part-time social service job. It paid six dollars an hour. But at least it was something. I fought not to feel useless and lost.

One day I drove to work listening to the news on the radio. I had the immediate sensation that I couldn't take in what I'd heard. The announcer said that Gene Segro was dead. Shot dead by a student, that morning in the cafeteria. It was horrifying, beyond comprehension, unreal.

Gene Segro was the principal of Dan's school. I had also worked for him as a substitute. I knew him and he was my husband's boss. It was 9 a.m. and he'd been murdered almost an hour before. The boy was dead as well. For reasons unknown then and still, the boy had shot Gene and then killed himself.

I was living the entire scene, all the while driving my car. Principals don't belong on the cafeteria floor, I was thinking. Their blood isn't supposed to spray on the walls. Gene Segro was a truly nice man, a generous man who cared about the kids. He was not supposed to have a crimson hole in his chest. He was not supposed to die during early morning cafeteria duty. It wasn't what happened at school. It wasn't what happened to a good man, a man that Dan and I knew.

The world around me was rocking. By the time I got to work I was a mess. I excused myself and went to the restroom. I was shaking and crying, rocking back and forth, my arms holding my shoulders. There were deep moans coming from my throat. I was in the depths of such deep grief I didn't know what to think. I was shocked by what had happened and I cared but even in the midst of my mourning it seemed out of proportion to me. Still I couldn't stop. I was relieved when Dan came to the office and we went home.

I didn't know it but I had begun the deepest spiral of all. I still don't know why Gene's death – or the manner of his death – hit me so hard. Maybe it was an accumulation of the disappointments and stress of several years. I was in depression and didn't see it. I was, in fact, having post-traumatic stress disorder, of which depression is a large part. So are suicidal thoughts.

A few weeks passed and I spiraled down even more. A Friday night came and all I could do was cry. I went to sleep for the entire weekend, waking for brief moments and going back to bed. On Monday morning, "it" was there. I wanted to die.

I don't think any words are adequate to describe what the wish to die is like. It is not a pity party. It is not even depression, although it is very much a part and product of it. But in many ways it stands alone. The urge is there as strongly and as unquestioningly as the desire to have sex. It is not logical or rational or even grossly overemotional. It just is, with a surety that the only way out is to follow its path. No other solution will end the pain.

I've heard many comments from people shocked and horrified by a suicide death. One of the most common is: "How could they do it? It's such a selfish act. How could they do it to the people they left behind?"

It's a very good question but it doesn't have a satisfactory answer. I liken it to what a person Is like during a diabetic low sugar attack. Sugar is needed in the blood to provide energy, not only to the muscles but to the brain. Someone in the throes of a seriously low sugar attack literally cannot think or judge. There isn't enough sugar going to the brain to allow the cells to do their work. Logic shuts down. Awareness shuts down. Judgment becomes all but impossible.

Being a diabetic, I know of this firsthand. The nature of these attacks, although unrelated to depression, come as close as I can get to describing what also happens in suicidal thoughts.

Although suicidal thinking has probably nothing to do with the amount of sugar getting to the brain, some of the same things occur. Logic, rational awareness, clear thought and judgment disappear. Something foreign takes over, something that outside of suicidal thinking doesn't even exist. In the film "Dead Poets Society," a scene depicts one of the characters just before a suicidal act. The camera loses focus. Strange, disturbed chords of music play in the background.

Everything freezes. It's not a realistic depiction of pre-suicide but it comes close in dramatizing it, because it is an otherwordly place, and it is an otherworldly act. When I reached that place – and have sometimes reached it since - I don't think about how my actions would hurt others, or how I'd miss the ones I would leave behind. I can't. The times I am capable of such thoughts I am not actually suicidal. Thinking about suicide and being suicidal are two different things.

Being actually suicidal takes place in a mind unrecognizable to its owner. When it happened to me that day, my thoughts become of one purpose only. There was no capacity to think of anything else or anybody else; nothing else could get in. It's not an explainable mind-set because the mind is not acting as it does in anything else. It is a dark and deep Antarctica, a place of frozen feeling and cold, robot hands that reach without mercy – for pills, for a gun or a knife. When I was there, it was as if the world had stopped spinning on its axis. I could not have been more cold and stilled.

On Monday morning I was at the zenith when some buried spark lit. It was enough to slow down the scary momentum. I drove to work like a zombie, feeling deeply afraid and ready to ask for help. I called my psychiatrist immediately. Ten minutes later I had a bed in the hospital and I was a patient in the psych ward – again.

It had been over thirty years since I'd been a patient in a psych ward. I thought I had gotten *way* past such situations such as this. As the education director at the agency I'd been the Answer Lady. I was the one who "knew" all about mental illness and mental health. I got the phone calls, I wrote the column, I made the speeches, and I was the one people asked. How could I now be a mental patient?

To make matters more difficult, many of the staff in the ward knew who I was. Some I had worked with at meetings and such, others knew me by reputation. I was very embarrassed. I taught others that mental disorders could reoccur or take different shapes, but as far as I was concerned, I was set for life. I was as loony as I was going to be, as controlled on medication as I could get. I had firmly decided that was all there was to it.

Being in the psych ward meant my worst fears became real. I wasn't better or holding, I was at the edge of the yawning black pit. I had no idea how to deal with it. I had lost my identity as The Teacher, I had lost my identity as the Answer Lady and now I had lost my identity, period.

I was in the right place for my safety and for a rest. Most psych wards are designed to stabilize and when the patient is well again, they are back on the street. I didn't expect any miracles; I just needed to be where I didn't have to pretend I hadn't "lost" it.

This particular psych ward offered little other than the opportunity to rest. Unlike the ward in Cincinnati, which was outfitted with all kinds of distractions, this one had nothing but a room with a couch and chairs and a TV. Patients spent much of their time pacing the hallways or sleeping in their rooms. I was thrilled to have a comfortable hospital bed that made it easy for me to sit up and read a book. Our "therapy" was a daily group conference in which a therapist would lecture and most of the patients would sleep.

My fellow patients were much the same as my first batch of fellow mental patients had been. They were a mixture of people who functioned well along with some who didn't function at all. All of us were there, though, because something had driven us away from the world.

Despite all that I "know" and have myself experienced, I'm still shocked when I see someone go from relatively "normal" to no longer in their right mind. Mental illness is a real, operative dysfunction of the brain, rendering one mentally dysfunctional as any other organ not working well would render whatever it effected. It's all very cut and dried; surely we can understand it and accept. But seeing the process up close and personal can be an awesome and unsettling thing.

I have a severely bi-polar friend who is generally pleasant, witty and basically "normal." But last year he didn't take his meds. He changed into a raving creature that tore up the house and thought everyone was out to get him. When I tried to reason with him that he needed to go to the hospital his response was "You bet I have to, because it's all bullshit over here." Then he refused to go. I ended up having to call the police to take him there.

THE MYSTERY THAT BINDS ME STILL

When mental illness takes over the "person" inside practically vanishes. It is deeply startling. A teenager I knew, bright, fun, full of great ideas, saw demon faces in the hallway, which turned into a rush of water coming his way. Better meds were found for him and he was back to his old self. Then something went wrong and he was back with the demons again.

I have seen extraordinary recovery and hope. I have also seen backsliding and despair. If one is mentally ill, (unless it's a situational disorder, as depression can be) the illness is always there. Patience, a good doctor, cooperation, medications, support from those who love and care – all or any of these things can make all the difference in the world. In some cases, a medication is found and it stays one hundred percent effective in the same dosage for the rest of someone's life. But it's different with everyone. Sometimes it takes years to find the right treatment and/or medication. In few - but nonetheless some - cases, recovery comes little to not at all.

When someone you know slips into the darkness, it can look like instant Alzheimer's. The person you know may look familiar, but they're not there. That's when it gets truly heartbreaking.

In this pysch ward, despite the dullness, I had a surprise. I watched a young man pace up and down the hallway for several nights, a headphone screeching loud music all the time. He kept the headphones on even when he attempted to watch TV, which, being so restless, he never did for long. was puzzled by the headphones until my education-director self kicked in. He was probably schizophrenic, I realized, and his headphones were a desperate attempt to keep the voices out.

One night the young man approached me. I recognized him instantly. "Hi, Ms. Singer," he said, "remember me?"

I remembered him. He and I had had a long, tangled, but ultimately happy relationship when he was my tenth grade student. He was so combatant that even I, having been a combatant high school student myself, could not relate. He was just a pain in my ass. His behavior was bizarre, too. He was constantly in trouble, not just with me but with other teachers and especially the assistant principal.

One day he told me he hated my class. Alright, I told him, let's talk about it. We did and for a long time afterward we talked about a lot of things. We got closer and friendlier and I was just working on understanding him when he walked out of school one day and never came back.

Now he sat across from me in this bleak place. I had been right - he told me he was schizophrenic. And all those years while he was punished and disliked, none of us knew what was really going on. I can't imagine any teacher expecting reasonable behavior out of a student literally battling inner demons, voices echoing unceasing in his head. But we didn't know. And my heart went out to him. He was still among us; he hadn't submitted to the suicide his voices advised. This "bad kid" was brave, braver than I could be. I'm not sure how long I could handle those headphones. But he just kept on keeping on.

And there we were, teacher and student no more; just equals in the loony bin. He was about to be transferred to the state mental hospital. Seven months later, I was hired to present a two hour workshop at that same hospital – the topic they assigned me was "I Am A Survivor Of Mental Illness." Sometimes the world is just a very funny place.

All told, the ward wasn't much but it kept me alive and safe. Also, I had free meals and got to see visitors. With full symbolic awareness, I was sprung on the 4th of July.

This time, my "going home" papers had a totally new disorder written on the front page. "Adjustment disorder," it read. Surprisingly, I didn't know what it was,

"It means you can't cope," said the doctor. "It means you can't handle stress."

I wasn't about to accept a sixth disorder. I decided it meant I would be a little weak for a little while and would spring up strong as ever after I had a little rest.

As it happens, adjustment disorder hasn't proved temporary at all.

Any time something scared me, denial was the first place I'd go. I stayed in denial about adjustment disorder for over two years. It was not only temporary, I believed, it was a sign of emotional weakness and when I got strong enough it would stop. The only question was how was I going to whip myself into shape? Nothing I tried seemed to bring about my promised strength. Instead, my mind employed whips and chains; I beat myself over and over again.

Tears were shed over how I "used to be" and was no more. I wasn't capable. I couldn't sleep. My hands shook more than ever. I put on more weight. I wasn't bringing in enough money. I was useless. On and on and on.

I knew better, of course. I knew that mental disorders had nothing whatever to do with emotional weakness. But the way I had changed was absolutely unacceptable to me. In the past I could be in the throes of whatever but if I ran into any stress, my philosophy was "bring it on." It was important to me, showing all how well I handled it.

The only thing I could think to do was to try. Anything. So I took a job in a convenience store. I was fired after two weeks. They said it was because I couldn't count. Well, I *can't* count, but I think it was really because I couldn't get the cigarettes to the customers fast enough.

I was trying to heal, but I couldn't figure out from what. I was also reeling from shock. I didn't feel strong at all anymore. I was naked without a reputation or a job. I had lived my whole life based on being a star. A star in a play, a star teacher, a star writer, a star storyteller, whatever. I had to be well known. Either my picture was in the paper, or I was writing in the paper. And now – I was nobody at all.

THE MYSTERY THAT BINDS ME STILL

The most frightening thing about being stripped of stardom is that all that was left was me – no masks and no trimmings. Not even as the poster child for the mentally ill.

I thought of it as spiraling down, but it was actually a journey. It took me down an entirely new path. If I was going to be no one but myself, I had to accept the whole, instead of just the pieces, of what that was.

With all the self-examination I had engaged in, at fifty I had to get out the microscope again. It hurt like hell.

Then, in October I went on another leg of the journey – quite literally.

There was a problem I had for years with pain in my legs and back. It had become much worse. It hurt to the point that I had to stop and rest every couple of steps I took. A friend of mine, greatly concerned, took me to her chiropractor, who performed various gyrations upon me and asked that I return that night. Later on there were more gyrations and some instructions as well.

"When you're ready to sleep," said the chiropractor, "lie on the floor on your back and put your legs up on the couch."

I did exactly what he said. Initially, it felt pretty good. But in the morning, when I woke up, I could no longer walk.

And it hurt like a son of a bitch.

I was hospitalized again, this time to await back surgery. Afterwards I was in rehab. I don't remember much from that time, but I know I was heavily drugged. I do recall talking to a number of people who weren't there but I felt obligated to talk to them just the same. One conversation was particularly boring so when I saw that my companion didn't exist I was relieved. I changed the topic of conversation.

I also recall I sang a lot. A *lot.* When Dan came over he'd wheel me into the various patients' rooms so I could take requests. I was astounded by the amount of lyrics flying out of me because I could have sworn I didn't know half of those songs. I sang to the doctors and I sang to the nurses and I sang to the physical therapists. I bet they miss me to this day.

Coming home, however, wasn't much fun. I would be home alone (except for weekends) for almost four months. I couldn't drive a car so I couldn't get anywhere unless someone took me, which I wasn't allowed to do for quite a while. I had to get up the stairs to the bathroom and I had to manage fixing lunch, etc. It was hard, inconvenient, aggravating and lonely and it *still* hurt like a son of a bitch.

Now I was truly broken, mind, body and spirit. My spine had grown into the shape of an S; my upper back was full of arthritis. Instead of feeling like my fifties had begun the next part of my life, I felt like the good and useful parts of my life were forever gone.

Maybe it was melodramatic, but it didn't feel so for me.

Eventually, love, patience and time have allowed some of my perspective to change. Yes, there are valuable things in my life that have been taken away. My body hurts. I can't work fulltime, I can't deal with much stress; I can't sleep. My spirit hasn't always hung on.

But on my better days I can accept it with more grace. I am neither unique nor alone. Everyone has difficulties with their bodies, some earlier than others. Everyone has things they could do and then can't. All of us endure strains and stresses and tragedies. I don't know what will continue to develop in my new, unshaped life, but I am certain it will be something interesting.

"Adjustment disorder" is another name on the list, but it's still not what my life is about. I look for what I *can* do, based on what I'm capable of now. Mental illness is neither the alpha nor the omega of my life. Neither is my back.

I was asked once, if you could be without mental illness, would you choose to be? I didn't hesitate for an instant – "no way." These disorders have caused a lot of problems for me. They continue to, and they don't go away. But they have also given me many gifts. I have creativity, a unique perspective and a sensitivity I doubt I'd otherwise experience. There are times when I have enjoyed the madness, and there are times when others have as well.

I'm still in there. I can lose sight of that. "Depersonalization" still happens from time to time, that hideous, chilling feeling of detaching, of going away from everything I am and everything I recognize as myself. It's part of my mental illness; it reoccurs when I get completely overwhelmed and drenched with stress.

I prefer health to the hospital, so today I have learned some new coping skills. I yell at my depression. Not at me – at my depression. I tell it it's a liar and I tell it to go away. I tell it it isn't real, that it's a fake. I tell it I am stronger, and better, than it is – that I have a life, that I am loved, and I invite it to shrivel up and crawl back to hell.

Sometimes it works.

Sometimes, when I'm not so down that all I can do is sleep, I dance. Leaping, hopping and twirling around makes it hard for anxiety to hold on. Singing helps. So does the company of other people. The middle of the night is the hardest time of all. Sometimes I drive over to the local convenience store at 4 a.m. I sip some decaf coffee and chat with the all-night manager. It distracts me and occasionally it amuses him. It helps us both to get through the night.

I do what I have to and I do what I can. Mental illness is an invader. It's most definitely a part of who I am; but which part I couldn't say. It's not segmented; I couldn't fill in the appropriate lines if I was outlined in a coloring book. Some of what it has given me I choose; some I don't. But as long as I know that it isn't my heart – as long as I know that I have a center that isn't a place in the dark – then I can live another day, sometimes fully, sometimes not, but I keep on breathing. And that's always a treat.

On the days I cannot dance I still have one blessing and a gift. Curiosity. I want to know what the next moment is going to be like. I want to be around for the next day because there may be something new, or unexpected. There often is.

Stubbornness, anger, determination and curiosity have keep me around when it seems little else can. Depression is poison. It blocks out the good, it blocks out the sun, it blocks out the truth, and it blocks out God. It blocks out love. When your days are filled with rituals and panic, doubt, sadness and fear, nothing else seems possible and nothing else seems real.

Faith is glorious stuff. I use it whenever I can. But the truth is, there are times when I can't. Those are the times when sheer cussedness comes to hand. You can't live your life blaming yourself for not being happy when you're mentally ill, anymore than you can blame yourself for having trouble walking when you have MS. You do the best you can. The key is celebrating the good stuff and hanging on through the horror. How to do that is an individual as the person who does it.

For me hanging on to life is sometimes a matter of just doing it because I can. Doing it because it's so hard to; doing it because so much fights against my doing so; doing it to say "so there." Doing it because my father taught me to and I honor him. Doing it because Dan makes me laugh. Doing it so I can write this book.

And hoping that you'll do it, too. Because one way or another we're all in this together, mentally ill or not. And if you weren't here I'd be that much less for it – because we have just accomplished a small miracle. I was alive to write this sentence – and bless your heart, you were alive to read it.

THE MYSTERY THAT BINDS ME STILL

CHAPTER SEVENTEEN: MIGHT AS WELL DANCE

In my workshops and lectures I was always a tragic soul- riddled with mental illness, struggling through life. If I don't get my perspective in order I begin to feel like I was a series of illnesses briefly interrupted by happy things. This is not the case. I've had a life full of adventure and joy and love; I haven't lived conventionally and sometimes I broke the rules – I have had great fun, and I have paid for it too.

I haven't been "Surviving Mental Illness." I've been living my life, and that's not about illness – despite it all, it's been about joy.

There are a lot of things I've liked about my life. I have a full and joyful existence, quite apart from anything else. I am not always in the dark. I'm outrageous, whimsical, and worship nonsense. I have the capacity to deeply feel and love. If two roads converge, and one is straight and the other is full of curves and trees and vegetation, that's the one where I'll walk. I am deeply curious about everything – and I'm always heading into the direction of wonder. I like my ease at laughing, my loyalty and honesty, too. I value my playfulness and silliness and my freedom. Most of all, I appreciate that even with depression and lousy self-esteem, I can still like me.

If I can't say that – or even more importantly, know it – too much of the bad stuff I've said about me will fill in the blanks. I've always been a cheerleader for people appreciating and celebrating themselves. But I've done little to do the same for me. So I try to be my own cheerleader as well. Sometimes it works. Sometimes it doesn't. When it does It reminds me that I am not an illness. It helps me recognize that there really are things I am glad to do and be.

One of these is a devotee of mischief. Creating mischief has been a lifesaver for me. It's a way of knowing that I'm alive and kicking and doing more than just standing up and taking nourishment. My dad loved reading me "Winnie-the-Pooh" when I was a kid. His favorite part was when the forest creatures got together to make mischief. They'd say, "What can we do to amuse them today?" He swore that this was exactly what I did every day. He was right.

Thoreau wrote about following "a different drummer." I've been hearing that beat all my life. My favorite play is Herb Gardner's "A Thousand Clowns." It's about a wildly eccentric character named Murray and the cockeyed way he sees the world. One of my favorite parts is when he's being lectured by a social worker, who begs him to "come back to reality." Murray says okay, but he'll only go as a tourist.

It wasn't my line, but I feel exactly the same way.

I have toured reality. From my perspective, it's highly over rated. Reality is okay to visit, but I don't want to live there. Dictionaries define it as "what is real, accurate and true." I believe reality is simply what you want it to be. I don't bother with it much – it bogs me down. Dad taught me how to

THE MYSTERY THAT BINDS ME STILL

look for the little people, and I'm still doing it. Only partially do I live in the world of the nightly news. The rest is in the much realer land of the fairies.

Such ability *has* come from, in part, from my mental illness. The rest has come from my imagination, and that is the engine that feeds my life.

One of the different beats I follow is storytelling. I've always done it but I've been "professional" for the last twenty three years. I define "professional" as being paid for it and damn good at doing it. Although taking storytelling very seriously may seem like an oxymoron to some, there's more to it than creating a lively narrative. To tell a story is to breathe its bones. It is to be its voice. It is to be the living embodiment of the tale as only you can tell it, using all that you can, body, arms, voice, hands, face. It is a sacred and holy trust.

It is also a very simple thing.

It's not about being theatrical, or stuff like taking a class in mime. It's about telling somebody a story – one of the simplest and yet most powerful experiences we can share. Nothing needs to flash on the screen, no television set needs to be turned on. It is not entertainment or even ceremony; it's a gift.

That's the twenty five cent explanation. Whether people buy it or not doesn't really matter. It doesn't take profound understanding to like hearing a good, well told rip-roaring story. The thing that I think is important is realizing we need to hear them. Stories do a lot of good things. They stimulate thought and imagination. They are good training for focus and concentration. They keep our brains alive and encourage our sense of wonder. We need these things. Telling stories is a great way to get 'em.

I am often asked if I am telling a true story. I am always telling a true story. All stories are true because they're about what's really inside us, the things we feel but keep secret, the things that aren't the surface stuff.

When I tell stories I am transformed. Only part of me is still me. Most of me is given over to being a channel for the story. I am the interpreter for the story to come through. I may leave my own mark on it but my commitment is to give every part of the story its due.

Every time I learn a story I must work out how it will be told. If there is more than one character, I have to imagine what they are like, how they would sound. Most of the time, I don't have to think about it at all. The Hairy Man just pops out of me roaring in the most amazing sounds. I don't know how he got in there, but he's exactly what he needs to be. The Peculiar Such Thang wails for its tailbone at just the right pitch. Rapunzel sings her lost prince out of the woods so sweetly; her tears wash the thorns right out of his eyes. Best of all is the raucous voice of the spirited and strong-willed Princess Gazork.

Storytelling is true multi-tasking. I have to keep my eye on the audience too. I have to know how to engage them, how to get that one straying boy's attention. If I sense resistance from the audience I know just what to do – launch into The Boogie Woogie Three Bears Song, and most of the time they're sold. I love pulling an audience into Story's special world. If I do it right, we're not in Kansas anymore.

My favorite storytelling session of all was the day I told stories to Amish children in their one-room school. I had the rare opportunity to be there because my friend Susan taught there. It was like being in another century. Some of the kids could only speak German; the older kids taught them how to speak English. They were all dressed in common Amish clothing, but some had plain black shoes and some of them with more liberal parents had sneakers on their feet.

None of them were used to video games or television. Most of them had never seen such things. They knew how to be still – not just with their bodies, but with their minds. They were fascinated. Their eyes popped and their mouths opened wide. Their surrender to the stories was complete. It was transcendent and it was spiritual. It was unlike any storytelling experience I'd had before or have had since.

My second favorite was the time I was a speaker at a juvenile jail. I had a group of tough, angry young men and I was supposed to tell them about mental illness. It was obvious they weren't in the least bit interested in listening. I offered to sing and tell stories instead. To my surprise, they were game.

To cut through their toughness I began by telling them I was going to sing a tender, gentle lullaby my mother used to sing to me when I was in my crib. As I expected, they looked at me as if I was a lunatic. Then I launched into a fervent version of "Love Potion Number Nine."

It made them laugh and they softened up. I told them a few more stories. It was almost time to leave when one of the boys raised his hand.

"You said you were going to sing us a lullaby and you haven't," he said. "We want to hear a lullaby."

I thought he was kidding and told him so, but the rest of the boys agreed. "We want a lullaby," they demanded and laid their heads down on their desks.

I was completely astonished, but deeply touched. I sang them a genuine gentle lullaby. Those tough thugs weren't so bloody tough. They wanted nurturing, just like we all do, and they got it that day. So did I.

Another golden moment was the call I got from a woman in New York. It was an afternoon, mid-week call – a time when telephone solicitors would often phone. The woman introduced herself as working for Henson Associates. I thought she was probably calling to sell me soap or something and I almost hung up.

She said, "Do you know what Henson Associates is?"

"No," I said.

"Well," she replied, "have you ever heard of Jim Henson and the Muppets?"

I was totally not cool. I screamed. "Why are you calling *me*?"

THE MYSTERY THAT BINDS ME STILL

I was one of several storytellers in the Eastern regional area that she was calling, she explained. Jim Henson was developing a show called "The Storyteller." He wanted to get background on every aspect of storytelling that he could. I wrote a seven page letter, packing in everything I knew and had experienced about storytelling. I got a letter back – telling me that my information was the best they had received and they wanted me to come tell stories to Henson and his staff.

Boy was I thrilled. Unfortunately, it didn't happen - for no reason I know of, and who knows what got in the way. But it makes for a glorious memory.

The more my imagination rambles, the more fun I have. Reality, for instance, hasn't gotten in the way of my becoming a princess and a queen. I have fantasized that I was a princess since I was a little girl. In my forties I found a way to solve the problem of how to finally become a princess and reveal my position in public. I simply began referring to myself as "Princess Mickie of York." When I teach summer classes in fantasy fiction for little kids, that's what they call me. I also use it in my storytelling, when I enter restaurants, and anytime I want to tweak an unexpected response. No one can tell me I'm not a princess. I also have a large collection of crowns.

I happen to be deeply in love with pumpkins, which I regard as magical fruit. Growing up in the city I never saw a pumpkin field. The first time I did I was as a young adult. I went mad with joy. I have longed to be the Pumpkin Queen. So Dan's daughter made me a pumpkin covered cape and an orange crown, and declared me so. That was title number two.

On the last day I taught, my students provided me with a cape, a sash and a crown. This time I was declared Queen of the Universe. They did this because when things weren't right I'd tell them it would all change when I became Queen of the Universe. That was title number three.

The fourth title, of course, was when I was made Fairy Queen at the annual Fairy Festival. This was very nice but I had little contact with my subjects, which kind of bummed me out.

I feel empowered any time I create something that wasn't there before. This can includes stories, people, decorating my house with stars and moons and suns - or putting together a dollhouse, cooking an original recipe, introducing a friend to someone else. Creating new universes is what has compelled me to paint murals on garage doors (with the owner's permission – and with payment, of course.). Sometimes I paint furniture, too. I like an unusual canvas – especially one like a two-car garage, so big it sprawls.

IAlthough I still have limited capacity to forgive, I can do it sometimes.

For instance in regards to The Prince. He knew not what he did; he was grasping at straws. He didn't want to be married and he didn't want to be alone. He still loved me but he didn't have the capacity to be with me. Before he got depressed he was a very different person – absolutely non-abusive and quite lovable. His illness and addiction had bottomed him out. We couldn't make it right. But we've remained pleasant to one another and made great effort to still function as David's parents. I speak with him very rarely now, but I felt good when he called me once to tell me had reached a goal. I knew it was important to him – and I was glad for him. I wish him the best.

Mom was the hardest of all. I've tried to tell the truth throughout this book, so I'm going to come out and say it. As much as there were neurotic episodes and craziness as well as regular mother-daughter stuff, there was something more. It was something sick, that even to this day, clutches my stomach when I think of it. First of all, from the time I was a little girl, Mom treated me as if I was a rival for Dad's attention – sexually and all. She regarded me as competition in everything. When she encouraged me to do things and praised me, she worked at finding found ways to bring me down, both in self-esteem, and into the waiting darkness. For me, she had rather the aspect of a witch. I found her literally scary.

And here's the reason why I was most truly scared – I have never admitted this publicly but here goes. I always had the distinct feeling that Mom wanted me dead. All her messages were death messages – "you were supposed to be a miscarriage," "don't worry, the walls will fall in," "don't ask your father to climb up the stairs to kiss you goodnight; he has a bad heart," "let's face it, you almost killed your father," "I'm going to kill you, Mickie," and so on. She was dying; Dad was dying, on and on. She predicted that I would get raped; also, if I had consensual sex, I would go crazy. Old men lurked everywhere, hoping to ravage me. She was a hypochondriac – she was sure she had all kinds of diseases, described them to me, and then I had them too. She called herself "an emotional cripple." She had no good news in her – and it scared me to death. I stayed away from her as much as I could.

There was more, and it's gut instinct stuff. Mom never came out and said it but I got the feeling that she wanted me to commit suicide. I had the impression that if I would do that, it would fulfill something Mom was looking for. What, I don't know. Proof that the world is a horrible place? Relief because her competitor was gone? I don't know. That was the scariest of all.

But here's the thing. Mom was in the hospital wing of the nursing home in Cincinnati. Dad had died. She had had a stroke. When I walked in she called out my name with such joy it made me cry. She was crying, too. After lunch, Mom was carefully laid in a hospital bed. I asked if I could get her anything. She said yes, a can of Coke. I brought it to her hand which curled around a non-existent coke, which she brought up to her lips and sipped. That was the most dramatic experience I had ever seen that when the brain is misfiring it "looks crazy."

At that time I was just a few months past my diagnosis at Johns Hopkins. I had meditated upon some of the similarities between Mom and I.

THE MYSTERY THAT BINDS ME STILL

I realized that she had been mentally ill in a time when there was little help available. The hurt she inflicted upon me came from her illness, not from her. Deep inside her there was a mom who really loved me. And I wanted to reach out to that mother and let her know I loved her, too.

I took Mom's hand and said "Mom I forgive you." We held each other and cried, and no other words were said.

Life with Mom was often awful. But it had its moments, too. The main thing I want to relate to is her love. She is the woman who made handmade Halloween costumes and potato latkes for Chanukah and found a way to send me to camp. She was doing her best. She couldn't help the other stuff.

Lately I wonder if Mom had a version of Munchausen's Syndrome by Proxy. Most women who have it express it through making their children sick. This gets them attention and feeds some need to believe in the negative always. I've never heard of psychological Munchausen's, but if it exists Mom may have had it. It would explain her peculiar darkness and her need for me to be crazy or dead.

It has unloaded a burden to forgive my mother... I hope that someday my son can forgive me as well.

One of my proudest moments was that I got my nerve up to leave Cincinnati. It was a very scary thing to do. I had strong attachments there both to people and places; I was 31 years old and I'd never lived anywhere else. I'd be leaving behind my brother and his family, of whom I was very fond. I'd especially miss the kids. My husband of the time (you know, The Prince) wanted to go back home, and home was Pennsylvania.

What concerned me the most was my mental health. I had no idea if I could handle such a big change. I couldn't imagine living without the warmth and support of my friends. I didn't know anybody there but his family. This proposal, I thought, was in the category of something I could never ever do.

I took a few days to feel about it, to think about it, and then I came to a surprising conclusion. I told The Prince: "Everybody has the right to have a new life at least once in their life. Let's go."

Here I am over twenty years later in this crazy, beautiful place. York County, PA. It is, for me, the best place to be and the worst place to be (apologies to Charles Dickens.) I am in the midst of the Bible Belt. Most of the folks who live here come from strict German tradition and families have lived here for years and years. The first influx of their coming goes back to the 1700's. Many of them still consider their identity to be Pennsylvania Dutch. It has been a very isolated place. The conservative ideas they have grown up with they hold dearly, as well as their traditions such as hunting and church going and living close to their families– and their conviction that as things go here, it is the same way everywhere.

THE MYSTERY THAT BINDS ME STILL

Some of the local folks aren't too wild about Jews or other minority groups. They disapprove of "making a fuss" which, one way or the other, I often do. Some can't imagine that people would think any differently then they do or believe there are other ways to behave. There are times when I am frustrated living here, and find it downright difficult.

That's the bad stuff. Here's the good:

Folks here are salt of the earth. They'll go out of their way to help anyone who is in need. Every time there's a family with a house that burned or a child who contracts leukemia or folks down on their luck who can't pay their bills, help is immediately on the way. There are spaghetti dinners and cut-a-thons and marathons and bake sales and basket bingo and anything, everything that will make it possible for unfortunates to get to a better place.

There are no city manners here - when people look at you, they *see* you. They appreciate who you are. When people meet going in different directions, someone will invariably step aside so the other one can pass. They are polite and they don't leave shopping carts all over the parking lots. If there's a line waiting at the ATM machines, there will be a long distance between the person at the machine and the one behind him. It's considered highly inappropriate to be privy to someone else's business where money is concerned. However, it is entirely appropriate, when not at an ATM, to know everybody's business in every other respect. York County has a small town atmosphere with all the pros and cons that brings.

I live now among vast acres of farmland and untouched woods. There are rivers and streams, mountains and the Appalachian Trail. The whole of the county is made up of swooping valleys and gently rolling hills. In all the time I've lived here I still feel like I'm on vacation. In the past I have seldom achieved serenity, but just being here often does it for me. If not every day, a countryside wander or sitting by a local stream gives me a pretty good facsimile. It is in many ways a place of peace, a place where one can begin again.

I also get a kick out of the many things that makes this area unique. I've never seen a place so devoted to food. There is no event that is not accompanied by tables heavy with baked goods and other regional foods. One can sup on whoopie pies, shoofly pie, and sugar cakes. Then there's chicken corn soup and boiled pot pie and snitz and knepp. It's all good stuff, and a lot of folks around here have the bodies to prove it.

I am intrigued by the language, too. In these parts, there is no verb "to be." The grass does not need to be cut; the shovel doesn't need to be put away. Instead, "the grass needs cut" and the shovel "needs put away." Also, no one seems to grasp the difference between "leave," "left," and "let." I hear "I left him take my coat." And "I left her go home." It really bothers me, though, when I hear "he let a message." It sounds like a fart.

THE MYSTERY THAT BINDS ME STILL

Being a very corny person I fit in here just fine. This is a place where it's major news when the strawberries come into season; it's in the newspapers and TV. Festivals and fairs are a constant, as are celebrations and parades. Bingo is very big. So are Elvis impersonators. People dress simply here – they're not into trying to impress. There are more church suppers than you can shake a stick at. Some of them are known to be particularly good. Personally, I never miss the crab cake feed at the neighboring Methodist Church.

Overall, I like what I've found here. I'm done with cities. Despite the drawbacks, I believe I'm in the right place.

Maybe in more ways than I think.

Because I know one thing: I've had so much fun there's no other way I'd ever choose to be. So take that, mental illness, and get into the back seat.

CHAPTER EIGHTEEN: L'CHAIM

That's pronounced lah-hi-em – it's a Hebrew phrase meaning "To Life!" It's also a popular Jewish toast made from the word "chai", meaning, of course, life. In Hebrew many of the letters also stand for numbers. The word "chai" stands for the number eighteen. Thus, this last chapter's name, since that's what this eighteenth chapter is about - how *does* one say "to life," especially when life feels like shit.

As it's expressed in the song, "L'Chaim," life is both bittersweet and sweet. Sometimes life is impossible and downright hell. How we humans keep upright and breathing through it all has always astounded me – but more so than that, it gives me a sense of awe. The human spirit is some pretty amazing stuff.

Holding out, celebrating, hanging on and snapping back – that's what it's about. To paraphrase a pretty clever fellow, there is a time for every purpose under heaven. But embracing that wisdom is the trick.

When I'm in a depressive cycle I am NOT celebrating, and I am not squeezing any lemons to make lemonade. I am not confident that "another day will come" and tomorrow will be better. One of the aspects of a mental illness is that your brain lies to you. Your perception is skewed; you are literally blocked from hope and faith. Often you are left with nothing but despair. Even when there's nothing to feel despair about. I am in depression and anxiety more times than not. Sometimes I believe my life can never be anything than sad and dark.

But I am stubborn and determined and that is what gives me strength. I rail and raise my fists and make a fuss. I stomp feet and kick ass and howl in the wind – whatever it takes. I'm Mack Singer's daughter and I don't give up.

Life is cyclical, and as surely as the bad stuff comes, so will the good. I was in my forties before my sense of things spiritual began to open up. I'm often long on doubt and short on prayer. But I am blessed with anger. It's my fuel. From it I draw determination: I *will* have a life, I *will* live it fully - because I *want* to. Even if that is as irrational as believing I can fly.

In an old Star Trek episode Captain Kirk was split in two, one half over-bearing and animal like and one half too weak to captain anymore. He needed that beast part to help him captain. They joined together and he became a healthy functioning Captain Kirk. I can relate. I am a very controlling person, for instance. But if I were not so I couldn't have been a teacher. Sometimes the darkness actually illuminates the light: If I don't see someone's shadow I'd have to believe them a vampire. I keep that in mind when I think I'm a "bad girl."

Sometimes it's okay to be in the dark.

Fear has always terrified me because I am afraid I'll never get out. It helps when I remember that even fear is a place to be. If the black pit is my home at least that's where I start. It doesn't have to be where I'll stay.

To paraphrase Ecclesiastes, "There's a time to build up and a time to break down. When I break down I feel lost. I can't imagine being able to climb my way back up. "Stoney End" is a song Laura Nyro wrote; hearing it always chilled me to the bone. It was about the end of me; the place from where I would never crawl out, forever surrounded, forever caught. The chorus scared me even more: "Mama, cradle me again." That's all I could hope for – a cradle to crawl in. A psychiatric ward.

But even when I don't believe it there *is* a time to build up. I've always followed Al-Anon's maxim, "fake it 'till you make it." It works.

If there is a time to everything and a time to every season there is a time for strength. There is also a time for the wisdom to know you won't always be strong. I always want try to stay with the strength, but doing so doesn't make me very wise. Another A-Anon maxim is "let go and let God." I hate it. But in the all the choice I'm free to make that is the only one I can't be free of.

Being alive I am entitled to all the joys and the horrors therein. If I say life is just wonderful, I'm an idiot. But if I say that my illness keeps me from having a life, I'm an idiot too.

The only thing I find amazing about miracles is when people don't believe in them. Sometimes we just don't recognize them. An ant – that tiny thing with its working body and strength and organized community – is a miracle. My son David is a miracle. Love is a miracle. Most of all, the human spirit is a miracle.

THE MYSTERY THAT BINDS ME STILL

Life has been far tougher for a lot of people than it's been for me. Surviving is a miracle. I don't believe we're never given more than we can handle. It sounds good, and it's reassuring, but I know firsthand that a human being can break. Sometimes it is *too much*. But it doesn't have to be the end.

Mental illness trains my brain in negative thought. It challenges my reality to believe in the good. So I grit my teeth and say "L'Chaim" anyway. Illness is only illness; it is not The Truth.

I'm curious to know – what's the next nifty thing that's going to happen? A free spaghetti dinner from Paesano's? A new friend to meet? A cup of perfect coffee? A neighbor's kids playing far into the night? Deer dashing into the woods? The sound of Dan coming home from work, his key turning in the door.... Being alive is full of moments like these, and they are, big and small, miracles.

They are the things to which I toast "To Life."

Even when life feels like crap.